Total Fitness for Women

Proven Strategies to Trim Down, Firm Up and Get Fit

Joe Luxbacher, Ph.D.;
Leslie Bonci, M.P.H, R.D.;
and Kim King, NSCA

Wish Publishing
Terre Haute, Indiana
www.wishpublishing.com

LCCN: 2001099360

The authors and the publisher assume no responsibility for any injury that may occur as a result of attempting to do any of the movements, techniques or exercises described in this book. These activities require strenuous physical activity and a physical examination is advisable before starting this or any other exercise activity.

Proofread by Heather Lowhorn
Editorial assistance provided by Natalie Chambers
Cover designed by Phil Velikan
Cover photo by Stockbyte, Picture Quest.
Interior artwork by Phil Velikan
Interior photography from Arttoday.com

Printed in the United States of America
10 9 8 7 6 5 4 3 2 1

Published in the United States by
Wish Publishing
P.O. Box 10337
Terre Haute, IN 47801, USA
www.wishpublishing.com

Distributed in the United States by
Cardinal Publishers Group
7301 Georgetown Road, Suite 118
Indianapolis, Indiana 46268
www.cardinalpub.com

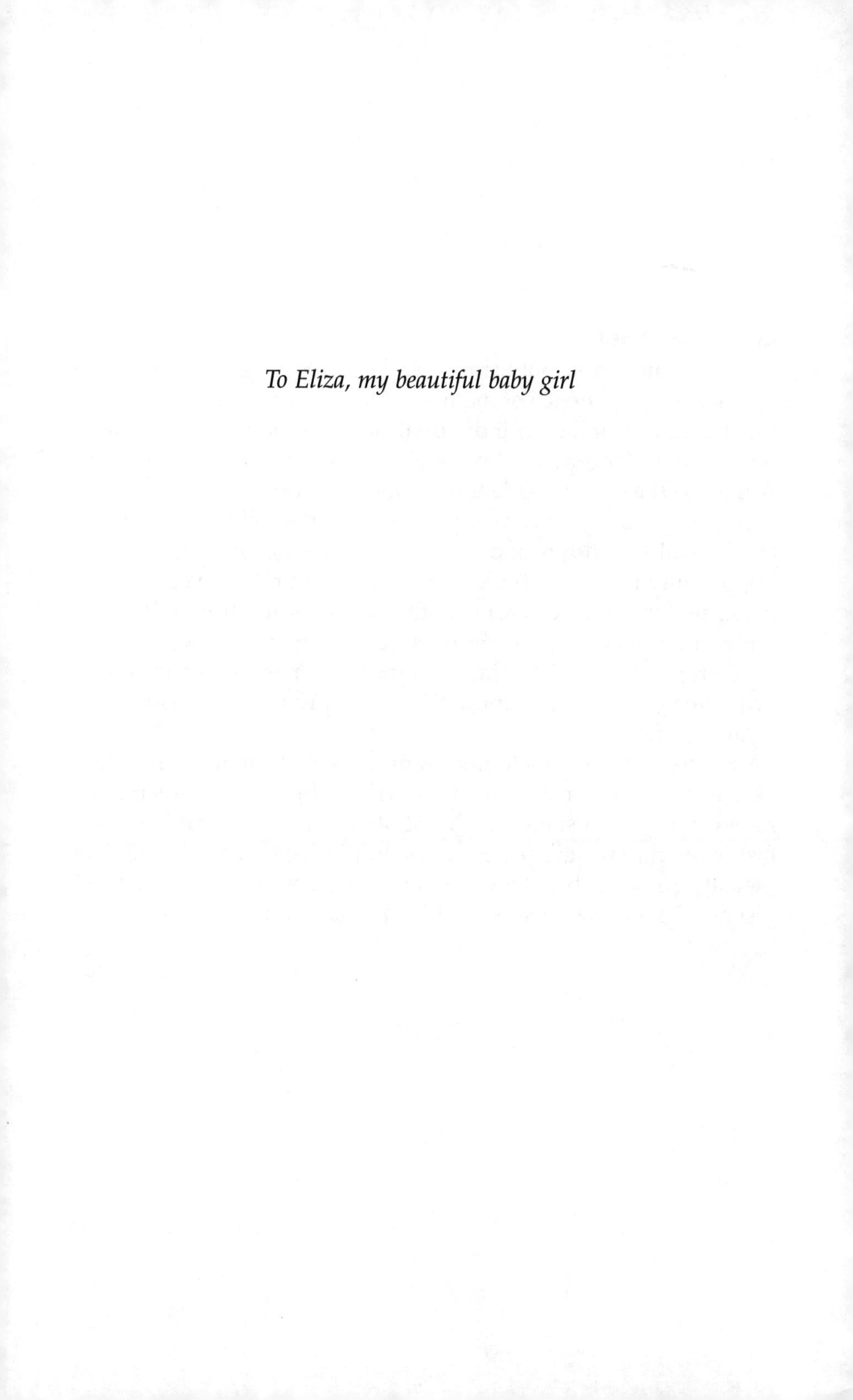

To Eliza, my beautiful baby girl

Acknowledgments

The writing and publishing of a book requires the support, cooperation and patience of many people. In that regard I am deeply indebted to a number of individuals for their help in transforming my original concept for this book into a completed manuscript. Although it is not possible to mention everyone by name, I would like to express my sincere appreciation to the following individuals. To Holly Kondras and Wish Publishing for providing me the opportunity to act on an idea and bring this project to completion; to Leslie Bonci and Kim King, both colleagues and friends, for their important contributions to the manuscript; and to Tony Salesi, physical therapist and athletic trainer at the University of Pittsburgh, for providing background information on the physiological assessment of human fitness.

Special thanks goes to my beautiful wife, Gail, for her willingness to sacrifice personal time for writing time and to tolerate the mood swings of a sometimes frustrated writer. Without her steadfast love and encouragement I would not have been able to complete the project. She, along with our children Eliza Gail and Travis Joseph, are a constant source of inspiration and happiness.

– Joe Luxbacher,
June, 2002

Table of Contents

Preface

For the better part of human history physical fitness and sport were considered exclusively a male domain. The underlying belief was that men were stronger and destined to be physical while women were weaker and more suited for a sedentary existence. Training for these roles began early in life. Boys were encouraged to be adventurous, active and athletic, to participate in all things physical. Girls were expected to play with dolls, to avoid sweat, to be at all times feminine. Young men were supposed to be competitive; young women cooperative. Physical activity and femininity were never mentioned in the same sentence. The few women who ventured into competitive sport did so knowing that they would be required to compete differently than their male counterparts. It wasn't until the 1960s that women were allowed to run any race longer than 800 meters, and they were forbidden to officially compete in the marathon until 1970. Such restrictions were based on notion that women were not physiologically and psychologically up to the challenge; that women could not compete physically on an equal basis with men.

Thankfully the times they are a changing. Today femininity and fitness are considered common bedfellows. It is universally accepted that women benefit from physical activity in much the same ways as men. Regular exercise makes women stronger, leaner, healthier, and in many cases, happier. We've seen firsthand that women, when provided the opportunity to participate and compete, can excel in a variety of traditional male events. Today's women are more physical than their mothers and grandmothers. They are running, playing soccer and lifting weights in greater numbers than ever before, and are far the better for it.

Total Fitness for Women has been written for today's active and soon-to-be active women. The information contained herein is appropriate for females of all ages and fitness levels, particularly for the millions who have struggled to lose inches and reshape their bodies. The chapters that follow will show you how to lose weight, redefine your physique, strengthen muscles and bones, and improve energy levels. Exhaustive workouts, starvation diets, and extreme self-denial aren't required parts of the program. Instead you will learn how to focus the collective power of skill, knowledge and attitude toward the realization of your fitness goals. You will be coached step-by-step through the process of developing and implementing a personalized program guaranteed to get results.

Section I discusses the many benefits that regular exercise has to offer and identifies potential pitfalls that prevent many women from achieving their fitness goals. Myths and misconceptions surrounding exercise and weight loss are examined and permanently laid to rest. You are introduced to the life-changing power of habit and are shown how you can harness that power to your advantage. **Section II** examines the cornerstones of total fitness — body composition, muscular fitness, aerobic fitness and flexibility — and explains how they combine to determine your present physical condition. **Section III** gets to the crux of the matter. You learn how to design a personalized workout plan by identifying your long-range targets and establishing the appropriate goals and objectives required to reach those targets. Proven strategies used to lose fat, strengthen and reshape muscles, improve aerobic capacity, and enhance flexibility are examined in detail. The truths and untruths about weight loss are revisited. Standard prescriptions used to improve muscular strength and cardiovascular fitness are examined. A variety of stretching exercises are provided. **Section IV** deals with special populations and extreme environmental conditions. Supplemental information is provided throughout the book in the form of tables, charts and sample programs. Important fitness-related issues are explored through the use of highlighted sidebars appropriately placed throughout the text.

The strategies provided in *Total Fitness for Women*, if put into practice, can effectively change the way you look and feel about yourself. Many of the principles can be applied successfully to other aspects of your life as well. I sincerely hope that you will put them to good use and wish you much success in your quest for lifelong health, fitness and physical well-being.

Joseph A. Luxbacher, Ph.D.

Section I
Becoming Fit: We Become What We Repeatedly Do

Habit is either the best of servants or the worst of masters.

– Nathaniel Emmons

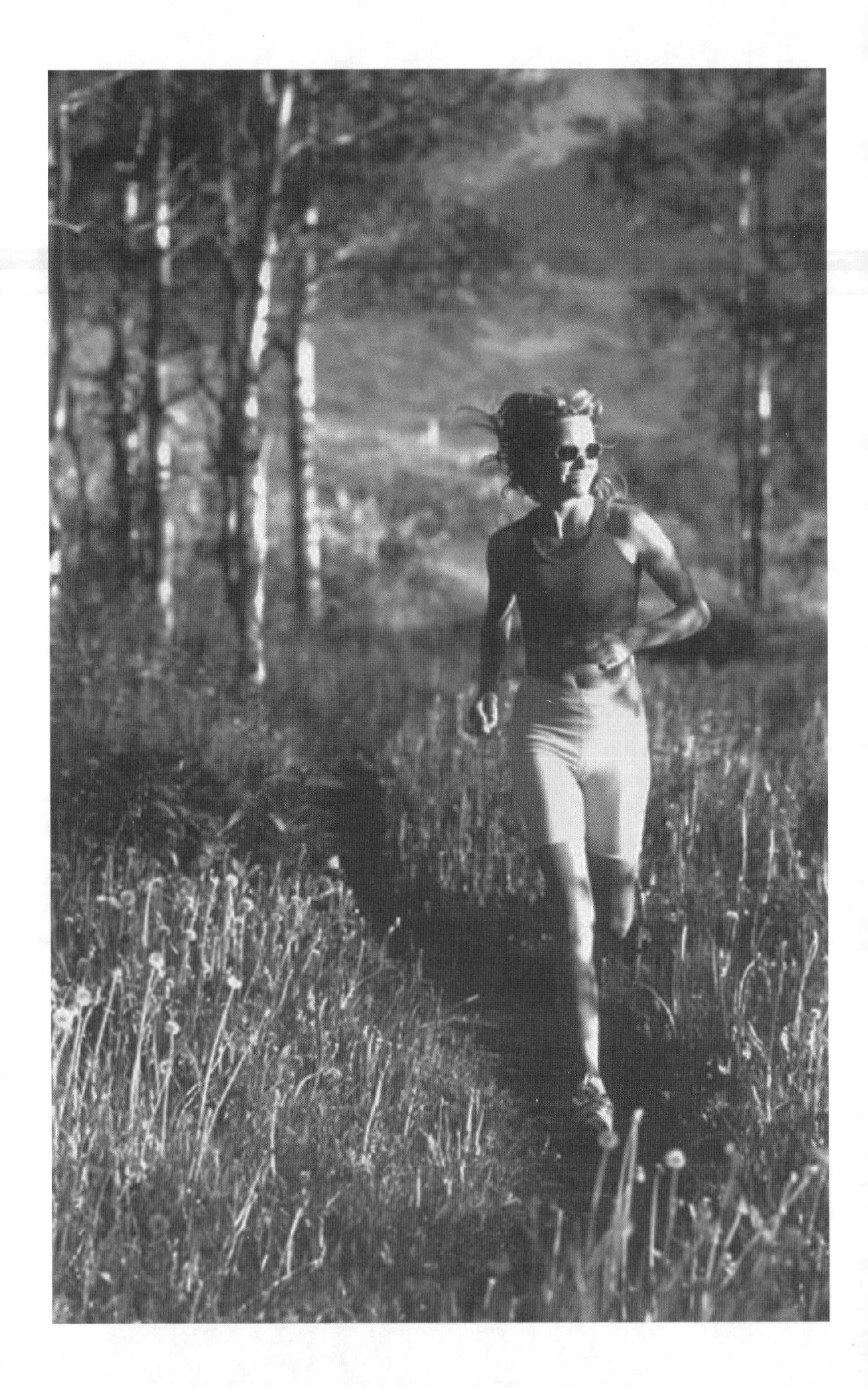

The Fit Lifestyle 1

The evidence is in and the verdict confirms what we've suspected all along. People of all races, young and old, rich and poor, female and male, will benefit from an active lifestyle. Even a moderate amount of physical activity can improve your health and overall quality of life. Regular exercise will reduce your risk of incurring coronary heart disease, high blood pressure, stroke, diabetes and some forms of cancer. It plays a vital role in maintaining body weight within healthy limits, an elusive goal for the tens of millions of overweight women who bounce from one diet plan to another with limited success. It improves mental health, reduces stress and helps to maintain healthy bones and joints. Last but certainly not least, a diet of regular exercise has been shown to slow and in some cases even reverse many of the physical changes commonly attributed to aging.

Despite all that we know with respect to the benefits of physical activity and exercise, plus the fact that our culture places high value on looking fit and feeling good, an alarming trend is taking place. Increasingly we are becoming a nation of the overweight and under fit. The numbers are frightening. Six of every 10 adults weigh too much for their own good. Nearly 40 million are obese — 30 pounds or more over a healthy weight. Sixteen million have diabetes, a leading cause of blindness, kidney failure and amputations. Fifty million suffer from high blood pressure, or hypertension. The dramatic rise in diabetes and hypertension over the past decade has been linked to an increased incidence of obesity, which is up more than 50% over the same period.

Contrary to what the multi-billion dollar diet industry would have you believe, overeating is not the primary reason for all the fat. Women today actually consume fewer calories than their grandmothers did. The real villain is an increasingly sedentary lifestyle. In short, there is an epidemic of inactivity going on! The following statistics, obtained from a cross-section of diverse age groups by the Centers for Disease Control and Prevention, illustrate this point...

* Fewer than one in five adults engage in vigorous physical activity (3 times per week for at least 20 minutes) during leisure time
* Only 20% of adults consistently participate (5 times a week for at least 30 minutes) in sustained physical activity of any intensity
* Approximately 1 in 4 adults report no physical activity whatsoever
* Inactivity is more prevalent among women than men, among older than younger adults, and among the less affluent than the more affluent.
* Only about 50% of people 12 to 21 years of age regularly participate in vigorous physical activity
* Levels of physical activity decline sharply as age or grade in school increases

While the short-term ramifications of these trends can be readily observed in our expanding hips and waistlines, the long-term effects are of greater concern. Our lack of movement is literally killing us. Low levels of physical activity have been linked to significant increases in death rate from all causes and have also been identified as a contributing factor in a number of degenerative diseases. Several forms of cancer have been tied either directly or indirectly to a total lack of physical activity. *The American College of Sports Medicine* estimates that our sedentary lifestyle is indirectly responsible for 250,000 premature deaths every year. That is nearly five times the number of people who die in automobile accidents. While most people would agree that driving without a seatbelt is hazardous to your health, it appears that the majority haven't been convinced that an aversion to exercise can be equally if not more dangerous.

Six Good Reasons to Exercise

Disease Prevention

Moderately-vigorous aerobic exercise performed on a regular basis will improve the ability of your heart and circulatory system to carry oxygen throughout the body. In effect your body becomes a more efficient machine that can better deal with the physical challenges of normal everyday life. Regular exercise also improves blood profile by reducing levels of harmful LDL cholesterol, a known risk factor for coronary heart disease, while at the same time raising HDL (the good cholesterol) levels. It will slow and in some cases reverse the buildup of fatty deposits in the coronary arteries. It decreases your chances of developing diabetes and hypertension. Last but not least, exercise can lower blood pressure in people who already have high blood pressure.

Weight Control

Regular exercise can play a defining role in winning your personal battle-of-the-bulge. Calorie-burning aerobic exercise promotes fat loss in the short-term. Muscle-building resistance training exercise promotes fat loss over the long term by elevating resting metabolism. Chapters 6, 11 and 12 discuss in greater detail the vital role that exercise plays in maintaining body weight within healthy limits.

Stress Management

Stress is a natural part of life. It can result from incidents as insignificant as sitting in a traffic jam to life-changing events such as the loss of a job or death of a loved one. A reasonable amount of stress isn't necessarily bad for us and in some instances may actually provide the kick in the pants we need to accomplish bigger and better things. Habitually high levels of stress are not good, however, and can signal the onset of heart disease, high blood pressure and poor mental health. Regular exercise has proven to be an effective means of reducing stress, feelings of depression and anxiety. A brisk walk around the block or workout in the weight room can release pent-up tension, take your mind off immediate problems and promote psychological well-being.

Strength

Athletes aren't the only people who benefit from strong muscles. Everyday activities like carrying out the garbage and picking up a toddler require a certain degree of strength. Strong muscles also increase the likelihood that you will be more physically active, if only for the simple reason that you can move about more easily, and make you less susceptible to injury and disability.

Range of Motion

An adequate level of flexibility is essential for long-term health and quality of life. Maintaining muscle suppleness and joint flexibility makes it more likely that you will remain physically active,

How Much Exercise Do You Need?

Because people exercise for a variety of reasons — to lose weight, gain strength, tone muscles, improve athletic performance — it is not possible to prescribe a minimum amount of exercise guaranteed to produce the desired results for everyone. It depends upon your level of fitness, short- and long-term exercise goals, orthopedic history and personal preferences. In terms of general health benefits, research suggests that the greatest gains actually come at the beginning of an exercise program, when you take that all important step from doing nothing to doing something. For most people consistency and duration of exercise are more important than intensity. Exercise-induced health benefits such as increased levels of HDL cholesterol and reduced blood pressure are directly proportional to the total amount of time spent exercising, and not necessarily related to how hard you workout. On the other hand, if your training goal is improved performance in a specific event (i.e, 10K race), then your workouts must be of greater intensity.

The American College of Sports Medicine (ACSM) and the Centers for Disease Control and Prevention recommend a minimum of 30 minutes or more of light- to moderate-intensity exercise on most days of the week. This standard is commonly referred to as the *exercise light* program. What constitutes light- to moderate-intensity exercise? Jogging, stair-climbing and cycling definitely fit the category, as do more functional activities such as brisk walking (three to four miles per hour), mowing the lawn and trimming the hedges.

also helps to minimize the aches and pains that sometimes accompany aging.

Strong Bones

A common malady affecting postmenopausal women is decreased bone mass and loss of bone strength. This condition, technically known as *osteoporosis*, is the primary cause of why older women are so susceptible to falls and fractures. Strength training coupled with weight-bearing aerobic exercise will stimulate greater bone density and, in turn, provide some protection against the debilitating effects of osteoporosis.

The Power of Habit 2

Habits are consistent, internalized behaviors that become an integral part of who we are and what we do. A steady diet of good habits applied to virtually any aspect of your life will, over time, lead to significant change for the better. On the other hand, when habits conflict with financial, physical or emotional goals you will be led down a road you'd really rather not travel. The ability of our habits to shape the future cannot be overstated, as they ultimately determine who we become and what we achieve. It's safe to say that good habits are a blessing while bad habits can be our downfall.

Becoming Fit

You need not undergo major lifestyle changes to generate major changes in your life. If you are willing to take small positive steps and apply these steps on a consistent basis, then you can achieve virtually all of your fitness goals. Guaranteed! We're not talking about extreme self-denial and discipline, marathon workouts, or starvation diets. Quite the contrary. The secret to becoming fit and staying fit is the development of habits that are congruent with your short- and long-term fitness goals. Three elements must be present in order to form a habit. **Knowledge** *(information)* informs you *what to do.* **Skill** *(strategy)* provides a framework for *how to do it.* **Attitude** *(motivation)* is a measure of your *willingness to do it* (See Figure 2.1). A habit will not form if one or more of these elements are absent.

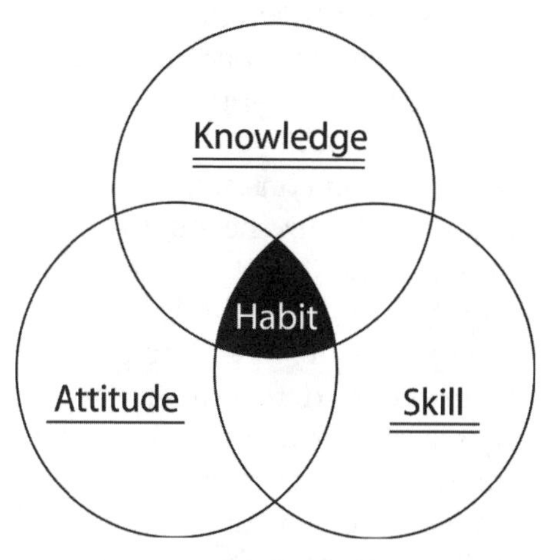

Figure 2.1: **Habits occur when knowledge, skill, and attitude overlap**

I'll attempt to illustrate how this works. Let's assume that you wish to lose a few pounds. You are very determined to lose the weight — you *want to do it (attitude).* You realize that to lose fat you must burn more calories than you consume over a period of time — you *know what to do (knowledge).* The problem is, you aren't sure how to go about doing it. You lack the necessary *skills.* You put your money on fad diets rather than sound weight loss strategies. You try very hard but receive very little in return. You eventually become frustrated, lose your motivation, and revert back to the lifestyle that got you overweight to begin with. You've failed to develop a new set of habits that will lead to long-term weight loss.

Harnessing the Power of Habit

The safest and surest way to achieve your fitness goals is to allow the power of habit to work in your favor. The following illustration focuses on one aspect of becoming fit — weight loss — and demonstrates how adopting a new set of habits can lead to huge payoffs down the road. Remember — you must know what to do, how to do it, and you must want to do it.

What to Do. There is a fundamental truism with respect to body weight. If you consistently take in more calories (energy) than are used to fuel daily needs, the extra calories will be stored as fat. If you consume fewer calories than needed you will gradually lose weight. One pound of body fat is the equivalent of approximately 3500 calories of stored energy. To lose a pound of fat you must create an energy deficit of similar magnitude. You can do this by eating less, exercising more, or preferably a combination of both. Once you've created a deficit of 3500 calories, whether it be over a period of days, weeks or months, you will have lost one pound of body fat. Keep in mind that the human body is amazingly sensitive to even slight imbalances in the *calories-in versus calories-out* equation. Increase your energy output by a mere 50 calories per day, the amount of calories it takes to walk briskly for 10 minutes, and you will lose five pounds of fat over the course of a year. Double the output and you will double the fat loss, assuming that calorie intake remains relatively constant over the same period of time.

How To Do It. There are myriad ways to increase energy output. Basically, you simply have to get your body moving. Get into the habit of performing any one of the following activities and you will burn approximately 100 extra calories.

* walk briskly for 20 minutes
* jog for 10 minutes
* clean windows for one-half hour
* skip rope for 10 minutes
* play tennis for 20 minutes
* shovel snow for 15 minutes
* rake leaves for 15 minutes
* swim leisurely for 20 minutes
* aerobic dance for 15 minutes
* wash the car
* mow the lawn for 20 minutes
* weed the garden for 25 minutes

You can attack fat from the opposite direction by reducing your energy intake. Rather than eliminating specific foods or food groups, get into the habit of substituting one behavior for another. For example ...

Instead of this ...	Substitute this ...
Three glasses of whole milk	Three glasses of 1% or 2% milk
Two pieces of toast, butter and jelly	Skip the butter
Large order of french fries	Large baked potato
Mashed potatoes and gravy	Mashed potatoes, pepper & salt
8 oz. of regular soda	8 oz. of unsweetened tea
Three cups of coffee, cream and sugar	Three cups of black coffee
One iced donut	One plain bagel
Two fried eggs	Two poached eggs
Pancakes with butter and syrup	Pancakes with light syrup
Pasta with cheese sauce	Pasta with marinara sauce
Canned fruit in sugar syrup	Fresh fruit
Pint of regular ice cream	Pint of sherbet or lite ice cream
Breaded chicken breast	Broiled, skinless chicken breast

Motivation to Do It. You should be buoyed by the realization that you can lose fat permanently and at the same time improve your body composition with a minimal amount of effort. You don't have to go on a semi-starvation diet or give up your favorite foods. You don't have to workout for hours on end. You simply have to make a few minor lifestyle changes. Become more physically active. Look for opportunities to burn additional calories. Make smart food choices. Eliminate nutritionally empty calories from your diet. These are not difficult things to do by any stretch of the imagination. Yet, over the long haul, they will lead to major changes in how you look and feel.

Inch by Inch It's A Cinch

When all is said and done, we are a product of our habits. The "little things" we do day-in and day-out rather than the "big things" we do once in a while ultimately determine our physical destiny. If you are presently overweight and out-of-shape, you won't be able to remedy the situation overnight. To arrive at a permanent solution will require that you scrutinize your eating and activity habits, and then make adjustments that are consistent with your lifestyle and long-term fitness goals. Focus on behavioral changes that you can live with. Develop a new set of habits. You probably won't see dramatic change during the first week or two of being the "new you," but be assured that you have initiated a process that will lead to positive and permanent physical change. All good things take time.

Building a Foundation 3

Becoming fit involves a collective mix of aerobics, nutrition and muscle-building exercises that when taken together create an overall effect greater than the sum of the individual parts. Fitness is not only about stronger muscles and a smaller bottom. It's just as important to improve those aspects not readily observable with the naked eye — elements such as blood profile, circulatory function, pumping ability of the heart, bone strength, energy levels, capacity to handle physical and mental stress, and immune function. To do so will require you to focus on day-to-day behaviors rather than the eventual outcomes of those behaviors. By embracing an active lifestyle you will automatically improve your inner self. The cosmetic benefits that accompany that improvement — toned muscles and a trimmer body — will take care of themselves.

Physical Fitness vs. Physical Activity

The terms *physical fitness* and *physical activity* are often used interchangeably, although by definition they are not one-and-the-same. Physical fitness is a performance-based concept that can be measured through the use of standardized fitness tests. How many push ups, sit-ups, pull-ups you can do, etc. In contrast, a classification of physically active reflects more on a person's lifestyle. Both physical activity and physical fitness are closely linked with good health, although it is entirely possible for an individual to perform well on a specific fitness test but not score highly on a general measure of good health. Likewise, the physically active person may not necessarily test well on a specific measure of physical fitness. Despite this apparent contradiction, the two are linked in the sense that being physically active will usually improve one or more aspects of physical fitness and, conversely, a high level of fitness makes it more likely that you will embrace an active lifestyle.

The Cornerstones of Total Fitness

Is the women who can run a 10K race in 45 minutes more or less fit than the football player who bench presses 400 pounds but can't jog a lap around the field without gasping for breath? And what of the national caliber 100-meter sprinter who struggles to swim a single lap around the pool? What does it really mean to be physically fit? From a practical point-of-view the concept of physical fitness encompasses of a number of interrelated components. Elite athletes training to develop a competitive edge must consider a wide range of parameters that include body composition, cardiorespiratory endurance, muscular strength, muscular endurance, flexibility, balance, coordination, speed, power, agility, mobility and nutrition. Those of us simply trying to improve our ability to successfully meet the physical challenges of everyday living should focus our efforts on the following:

- **Body composition** refers to the chemical makeup of the body or, more specifically, the relative amount of lean mass (muscle, bone, tissues and organs) to fat mass. This relationship is usually described in terms of *percent body fat*. A percent body fat of 25% automatically translates to a corresponding value of 75% lean mass. Body composition is one indicator of your level of fitness.
- **Cardiorespiratory (aerobic) fitness** relates to the body as a whole rather than isolated muscle groups, and is directly linked to the efficiency of the heart and circulatory system. A strong heart and healthy blood vessels will lower your risk of coronary heart disease, the #1 killer of American women. Aerobic exercise of sufficient frequency, duration and intensity will improve your body's ability to deliver nutrients to the tissues and remove unwanted waste products. Stamina will improve as your body becomes more efficient at providing the working muscles with oxygen. You will look and feel younger. The 45-year-old marathoner who cross country skis and plays tennis may be chronologically older than the 35-year old couch potato, but physiologically she is much younger.
- **Muscular fitness** has two primary components. *Strength* refers to the ability of a muscle or group of muscles to exert force for a brief period of time. *Endurance* is a measure of the ability of a muscle or group of muscles to sustain repeated contractions. Both strength and endurance can be improved through resistance (weight) training. In the not-

TABLE 3.1: Exercise Participation: What Women Are Up To

Women consitute a majority of participants in 14 of 62 fitness and recreational activities surveyed for 2000 by the National Sporting Goods Association. Here is what they like to do most:

Sport activity	*Total Participation (in millions)*	*Percentage female participants*
1. Step Aerobics	7.3	91.4%
2. Aerobics	19.6	75.4
3. Kickboxing	2.7	67.7
4. Exercise walking	50	63.9
5. Horseback riding	N/A	62.4
6. Roller skating	5.2	62
7. Ice skating	4.5	61.8
8. Volleyball	6.4	55.2
9. Swimming	30.8	54.7
10. Badminton	2.6	52.9
11. Calisthenics	6.6	52.7
12. Exercising w/Equipment	23.1	51.9
13. In-line skating	12.2	51.6
14. Cross country skiing	1.2	50.3

so-distant past weight training was considered strictly a "man thing." I can still recall the Charles Atlas ads of my youth showing a musclebound beach bully kicking sand on the skinny 97-pound weakling. To add insult to injury, the muscle guy got the girl as well! The fact that strength training can provide health-related benefits for women as well as men was largely overlooked. Today we know better. Women are lifting weights in record numbers and reaping the benefits.

✳ **Flexibility**, defined as the range of possible motion in a joint or series of joints and the surrounding muscles, provides the bridge that can take you from a sedentary existence to a high octane physically-active lifestyle. Maintaining an ad-

Fueling Exercise: The Ideal Mix?

The mixture of fuel used by the muscles depends upon how hard you are working. During light- and moderate-intensity exercise the muscles run on a mix of free fatty acids and glucose. As intensity increases fats become a less efficient energy source. Glycogen (stored sugar) becomes the preferred fuel for both short-term (sprint) and long-term (endurance) exercise. You can maximize glycogen stores by including a high percentage of carbohydrates in your diet. The type of carbohydrate consumed is not particularly important, as both complex (starches) and simple (sugars) carbohydrates are effective in increasing glycogen stores. For health reasons it is better to eat a greater percentage of nutrient-dense, complex carbohydrates such as pasta, rice, cereals, vegetables, and grains, as opposed to sweets and simple sugars.

equate level of flexibility, particularly as you get older, will enable you to move about more freely and makes movement more enjoyable. It also helps to prevent exercise-related injuries that can sidetrack your progress

- **Low-fat high-energy diets** include six essential nutrients. *Carbohydrates* are the sugars and starches found in foods such as breads, cereals, rice, potatoes, pasta, fruits, vegetables, milk and milk products. *Proteins* function primarily as building blocks for the growth and repair of cells. We obtain dietary protein mostly from animal sources such as meat, poultry, fish and dairy products, and to a lesser extent from vegetable sources such as beans and nuts. *Dietary fat* provides a very concentrated source of energy, about 9 calories per gram or 36 calories per teaspoon. We obtain fat primarily from meats, eggs, daily products, nuts and vegetable oils. Carbohydrates, proteins and fats all provide calories and therefore play a role in weight gain and loss.

  Vitamins are organic substances that perform metabolic functions within the cells. We obtain vitamins primarily from the foods we eat and through vitamin supplements. *Minerals* are inorganic compounds that occur freely in nature. We use minerals in a variety of ways, mostly to form various structures of the body and also to regulate chemical reactions within cells. We get our supply of minerals almost exclusively from the foods we eat and drink. *Water* makes up 60% to 75% of our body weight. Our body gets its supply of water from the foods we eat, the liquids we drink, and as a byproduct of energy yielding chemical reactions that occur in the body. From a nutritional point-of-view, we often take water for granted although, in reality, it is our lifeblood. While humans can survive for weeks without food, we can't do without water for more than a few days. Vitamins, minerals and water, each important in their own right, do not provide calories and therefore do not play a role in weight loss or gain. A more detailed discussion of nutrition can be found in Chapter 18.

Slim Down • Firm Up • Get Fit 4

Proven strategies for losing fat, building muscle, developing endurance and staying limber are grounded in universal physiological principles. No gimmicks or gadgets, just sound information that, if applied, will enable you to achieve your fitness goals. The following aspects of fitness are discussed in greater detail throughout the book. A brief introduction is provided here to provide you with a general idea of where we are going and how we plan to get there.

The Fundamentals

Fat Loss. If you are presently carrying too much fat it is because, over time, you've taken in more energy (calories) than was needed to meet daily requirements. The only proven way to lose the extra weight is to reverse the process. You can do this through modifications in your eating and exercise habits.

Building Muscle. You improve strength by pushing or pulling against a resistance greater than that to which your muscles are accustomed. The muscles gradually adapt to moving the increased weight by becoming stronger. As your strength improves a proportionally greater resistance will be required to stimulate additional gains.

Developing Endurance. You should consider four exercise factors — *mode, frequency, duration, and intensity* — when designing a program to improve aerobic endurance. Mode refers to the type (jogging, walking, biking, etc.) of exercise. Frequency, duration and intensity deal with how often, how long and how hard you exercise. To realize a conditioning effect you must exceed a minimum threshold for each factor.

Staying Limber. Women are, by nature, more flexible than men across all age groups. Even so, your range-of-motion will gradually decline with age unless you make a conscious effort to maintain it. Simple activities such as bending over to tie your shoes will become more difficult. Common, everyday movements will require more effort. In all likelihood you will become more sedentary, which will eventually lead to muscle loss, depressed metabolism and weight gain. Suffice to say, maintaining an adequate range of motion is important for sustaining the quality of life. Flexibility can be enhanced through a program of static stretch exercises.

Principles of Training

The following principles apply to all forms of physical training and will directly effect your efforts to become physically fit.

Specificity. Commonly referred to as the S.A.I.D. Principle *(Specific Adaptations to Imposed Demands)*, it states that your body will adapt in specific ways to the physical demands imposed upon it. In other words, to achieve a specific exercise outcome will require a specific exercise prescription. For that reason long-distance runners train differently than middle-distance runners who train differently than sprinters. Workouts will also vary depending upon your short- and long-term training goals. In a nutshell, there isn't one plan that fits all.

Overload. Although it is usually associated with strength training, the overload principle actually applies to all forms of physical conditioning. Simply stated, to develop strength you must overload the muscles beyond the point to which they are normally stressed. To improve aerobic endurance you must overload the cardiovascular system beyond the point to which it is normally accustomed. As your level of fitness improves you must increase the training load to stimulate further gains.

Progression. Attempting to do too much too soon will usually set you back. It is best to move forward in small steps rather than large leaps. Slow and steady will eventually win the race.

Hard-Easy-Hard. More is not always better. Your body will eventually break down if workouts are too hard, too long or too frequent. Our physiological systems require sufficient time to recover and regenerate after strenuous exercise. You will maximize training results by varying the nature and intensity of your workouts. Go hard one day, easier the next. You can also use a variety of exercises that stress the muscles in slightly different ways.

Reversibility (Disuse). Consistency of effort is a key to success in most every endeavor. Becoming fit is no different. If you exercise only occasionally, or stop entirely for extended periods of time, you reverse the process. The composition of your body will change for the worse. Levels of aerobic and muscular fitness gradually dissi-

The Natural Method of Becoming Fit

Crosstraining involves the use of a variety of exercises to develop a well-rounded fitness program. Most of us, although we did not realize it at the time, spent a good portion of our youth crosstraining. Our days were filled with riding bikes, climbing trees, playing ball, swimming at the local pool and mowing the lawn. Adults can adopt a similar philosophy to make workouts more interesting and enjoyable.

Serious crosstrainers balance their workouts between aerobic, strength and flexibility exercises. They also vary the exercises within each category. For example, aerobic workouts alternate between weight-bearing activities such as jogging and skipping rope and non-weight bearing exercises such as stationary cycling and swimming. Strength workouts can be organized in similar fashion. Use machines for a few weeks, then switch to free weights for the next cycle. As a change-of-pace do it the old fashioned way with a variety of push-ups, pull-ups, dips, sit-ups and crunches. A reasonable mix of exercise includes three or four days of aerobic training per week, two or three days of strength training and flexibility exercises every day or, at the least, every other day.

pate. Flexibility decreases. The principle of reversibility is sometimes referred to as the *use it or lose it* principle.

Individual Response to Training

Some things in life seem to defy logic. You would expect that two people who perform the same workout regimen would experience the same fitness gains. That doesn't always happen. Normal variation among individuals can explain in part why some people demonstrate greater improvement than others. It doesn't explain away all of the differences, however. The following factors also play a role in determining how well you will respond to a given exercise program.

Level of Fitness. The more out-of-shape you are at the beginning of an exercise program, the more rapidly you will see improvement. The most significant changes occur with people who go from doing nothing to doing something. As you become more fit you will have to work harder to stimulate continued improvement.

Physical Maturity. Maturity is closely linked with an individual's *state of readiness*, which in turn affects her ability to exercise. If two women follow the same workout plan but one is more physically mature and trains at a greater intensity relative to her level of fitness, then that individual will experience more dramatic gains.

Heredity. We inherit certain physical attributes that can impose limits on our potential for physical development. Heart and lung size, muscle fiber characteristics, skeletal structure and body type are a few such examples. Most of us never come anywhere close to reaching our physical limits, however, so if you exercise on a regular basis you will definitely see progress. It just might not be as fast as your workout partner.

Nutrition and Rest. Improvements in fitness are due in part to changes that occur on a cellular level. Oxygen carrying capacity (aerobic fitness) and muscular contractile ability (strength) are cases in point. Without proper nutrition and sufficient rest, such improvements will be diminished.

Barriers to Success 5

You won't achieve anything of value without an investment of time, effort, commitment and perseverence. This rule applies to virtually every aspect of our life, including physical fitness. The high exercise dropout rate (50+ percent) provides warning that you will encounter obstacles on the road to becoming fit. The majority are mental as opposed to physical in nature, and can be overcome or avoided entirely through simple attitudinal adjustments. Don't allow the following bumps in the road prevent you from realizing your fitness goals.

Short-term View. Many people begin a fitness program expecting a quick fix. They opt for extreme diets or radical workouts that promise dramatic change overnight. Be wary of such claims. Think about it. You didn't go to bed one evening toned and trim and wake up the next morning out-of-shape and overweight. The transformation from fit to unfit usually stretches over a period of months or even years. You cannot regain in a week or two what it took months or years to lose. It's OK to think big, but you've got to start small. Rome wasn't rebuilt in a day, and your body won't be either. It is a slow and steady process that requires a long-term commitment.

Misinformation and Myth. The fitness market is glutted with books, videos and infomercials claiming to know the secret of how to lose 30 pounds in 30 days or develop six-pack abs in 60 seconds a day. For a price they will even reveal the secret to you! Don't be misled by promotional hype and hoopla. When it comes to becoming fit there are no secrets! If the results promised from an exercise or diet plan sound too good to be true, they probably are.

Lack of Confidence. If previous efforts have come up short you may find it difficult to gear up for yet another try at it. That's only human nature. Take solace from the fact that in all probability your past failures were not due to an inherent character flaw or lack of effort. It's much more likely that your intentions were good, but your information was bad. As they say in the financial markets, past results do not dictate future performance. *If you know what to do, how to do it, and are willing to do it, then you can take control of your physical destiny.* That is what this book is all about.

Failure to Plan. Preparation is an essential part of every successful venture. You wouldn't think of building a house, saving for retirement, or even writing a book without first formulating a blueprint to guide your actions. A well-conceived plan will identify your targets, focus your efforts, and enable you to make the most efficient use of time and energy.

Procrastination. It is no secret that the first step is often the most difficult. It's also the most important because it sets the process in motion. This book is designed to take the uncertainty out of the "get fit" equation, to provide you with the knowledge and know-how needed to achieve your fitness goals. Along with that knowledge will come the confidence required to put the information to good use.

Fear of Failure. You've probably heard the bad news. Ninety-five percent of people who lose weight gain most or all of it back. More than half who begin an exercise program quit within the first three months. Why go through the hassle of planning and implementing a program that is ultimately destined to fail? For the simple reason that you will not fail unless you set yourself up for failure. The vast majority who have tried and failed did so because they chose to pursue a "quick fix" remedy rather than a long-term solution. It may have been a popular diet plan that required specific foods be eaten in specific combinations at specific times of the day, or a workout program that was simply too intense, too inconvenient, or too boring. In either case the program was destined for failure because the person couldn't live with it. The sooner you flush the quick fix mentality from your mind the better off you will be. Focus instead on a life-plan that takes into account your personal likes and dislikes, a program that fosters slow and steady progress toward the realization of your fitness goals.

Lack of Time. "I'm too busy" is the most oft-cited reason for not exercising regularly. Granted, surveys do show that Americans have less free time than ever before. We're working longer hours and taking fewer vacations. Schedules are tighter and less flexible. That being said, citing lack of time as the reason for not exercising is a pretty lame excuse. I say this for a couple of reasons. First, you don't have to exercise for hours on end to get results. We've already discussed how you can reap substantial health benefits by performing as little as 30 minutes of physical activity on most days of the week. Second, you have much more time than you think. Suppose that you exercise five times per week for a period of 30 minutes each session. Assuming that you sleep 8 hours per day, workouts would account for slightly more than 2% of your waking time. That is probably less time than you spend sitting in front of the TV. In most cases the actual problem is not a lack of time. It is poor time management!

Takes Too Much Effort. If you grew up playing competitive sports you probably had the phrase *"no pain, no gain"* imprinted on your psyche. Today we know that isn't the case. You don't have to exercise very long or very hard to realize positive fitness benefits. You merely have to do it on a regular basis.

Section II
Becoming Fit: The Essential Elements

Fitness can neither be bought nor bestowed.
Like honor, it must be earned.
– Anonymous

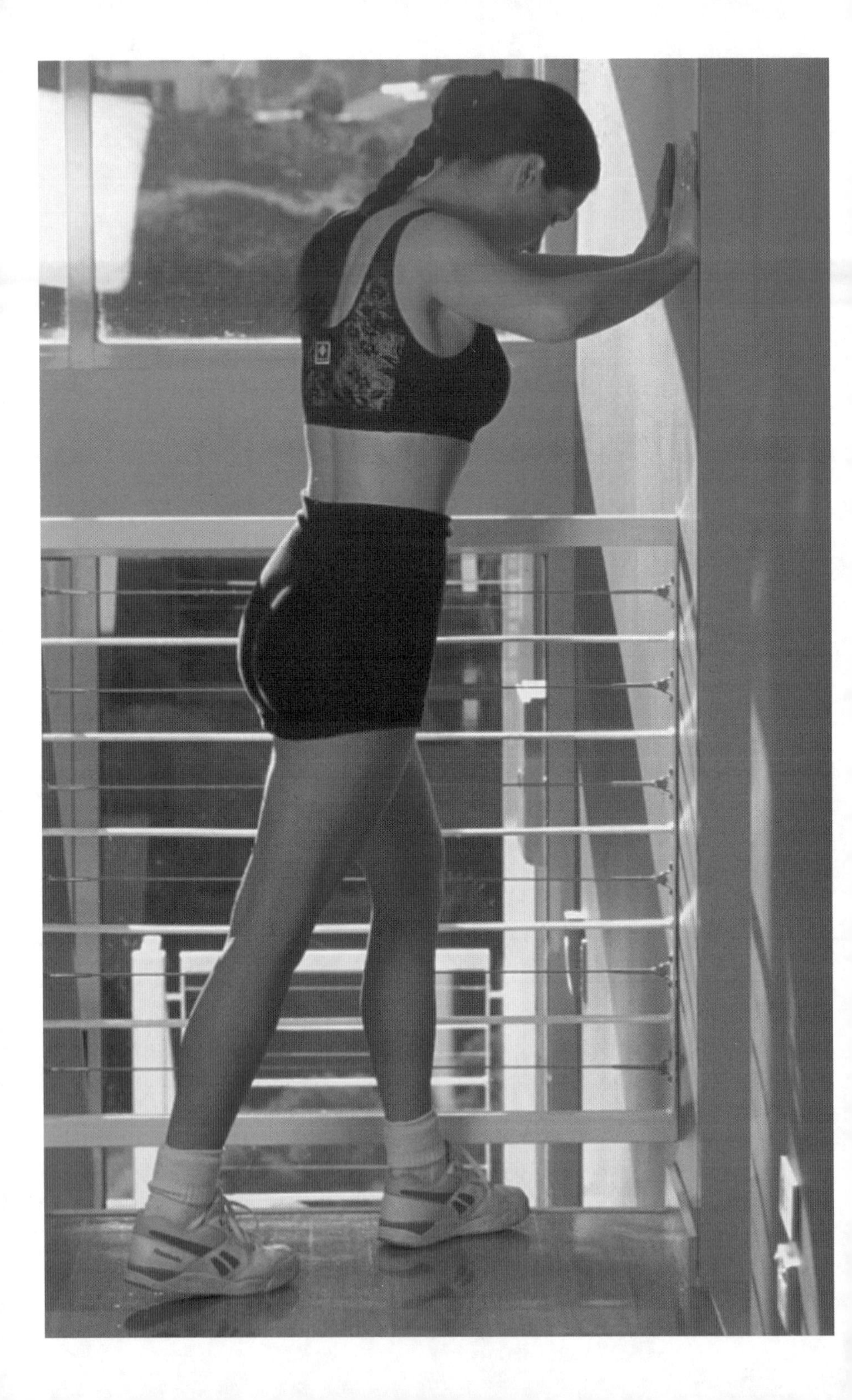

Body Composition 6

Your body is composed of two general categories of tissue: *fat-free (lean) tissue* which includes muscles, bones, organs and connective tissues, and *fat (adipose) tissue*. Body composition, commonly expressed in the form of *percent body fat*, refers to the relative percentages of lean mass and fat mass in relation to total body weight. A healthy body composition places you at a lower risk for coronary heart and artery disease, stroke, diabetes and hypertension, and makes it more likely that you will maintain an active lifestyle. Physical considerations aside, body composition is also important because it can influence self-concept. Many societies, including our own, place high value on a lean body appearance. Obesity, particularly in women and children, can contribute to a negative body image and poor self-concept.

Sifting Through the Terminology

The terms *overweight, over fat* and *obese* are often used interchangeably although they do not necessarily describe the same condition. By definition a woman is *overweight* if she weighs more than predicted for her age and height according to standard weight tables. Body weight ranges are based solely on population averages, and do not necessarily conform to ideal weight. (See Table 6.1) A woman is considered *over fat* if she is carrying more body fat than the national average for her age. The over fat individual is likely to be overweight as well, but not necessarily so. For example, a woman who is carrying a greater than average amount of body fat but a less than average amount of muscle mass may fall within the normal body weight range as defined by the height-weight charts. By definition she would be over fat but not overweight! A woman is considered *obese* when her total amount of body fat is equal to or greater than 35 percent of her body weight (25 percent for men). The health risks of obesity far exceed both the overweight and over fat conditions. A landmark study conducted by the American Cancer Society of more than one million Americans, the largest survey ever done on obesity and mortality, showed conclusively that obese people run a higher rate of premature death. The study found a clear link between excess weight and a higher risk of dying from heart disease and cancer. This trend was evident even among those who didn't smoke and were otherwise healthy.

Height-Weight Tables

Standard weight tables provide minimum, average and maximum weights (in pounds) for a given height, age, and sex. How helpful are these tables in determining an appropriate body weight, and what can they tell you specifically about your weight? The answer on both counts is mixed. According to insurance company statistics, desirable (normal) weights are associated with a longer life span. If you fall within the normal weight range specified for your height, age and sex, you are less likely to die a premature death. A body weight in excess of the predicted norm has greater health-related risks associated with it. For this reason insurance companies often charge a higher premium for individuals who are 20% or more above their predicted weight. A major limitation of standard age-height-weight tables is that they do not take into account the composition of a person's body.

TABLE 6.1: Desirable Weight for Women (Age 25 and above)

Height (without shoes)	Weight in lbs. (without clothes)
5′0″	103-115
5′1″	106-118
5′2″	109-122
5′3″	112-126
5′4″	116-131
5′5″	120-135
5′6″	124-139
5′7″	128-143
5′8″	132-147
5′9″	136-151
5′10″	140-155

These guidelines, issued by the Metropolitan Life Insurance Company in 1959, are recommended over more recent editions, which provide false reassurance to a large fraction of individuals who are not defined as overweight.

Energy Balance and Body Composition

The chemical makeup of your body is determined by a complex set of genetic and environmental factors. Although you can't do much to alter the genetic component, it is possible to effectively manage relative amounts of fat and muscle by manipulating certain environmental factors. Maintaining a healthy body composition is purely a matter of balancing the number of calories you consume with the number of calories you burn through normal metabolic processes and physical activity. The relationship between these two factors (*energy-in* vs. *energy-out*) is commonly referred to as your *energy balance.*

Metabolism refers to the energy used daily to keep your body functioning normally. To a large extent metabolism is genetically programed and can vary significantly from one person to another. Some people naturally require more energy than others just to keep their body running smoothly. We refer to these individuals as having a *high metabolism* because their engine always seems to be running in high gear. They eat anything and everything and don't gain weight. Those of us who possess a slower metabolism require fewer calories to keep us going and as a result may have a more difficult time maintaining normal body weight. Metabolic rate is under the control of various hormones and is not easily altered in the short-term. There are, however, a few simple strategies that you can implement to rev up your calorie-burning furnaces (See Chapter 12).

The Science of Weight Gain and Loss

The *First Law of Thermodynamics* states that energy can neither be created nor destroyed, although it can be changed in form. This fundamental law of physics provides the answer to why people gain weight. A *positive energy balance* exists when energy (calorie) intake exceeds energy expenditure. The extra calories are not lost or destroyed, but instead are converted to body fat and stored beneath the skin and within the muscles. Over a period of time a positive energy balance can lead to substantial fat gain. A *negative energy balance* exists when, on average, calorie intake does not meet energy requirements. Your body gets the extra energy it needs by converting stored body fat. As a result, you gradually lose weight.

It is important to consider that weight loss (in pounds) does not automatically equal fat loss. The composition of the loss will

3000 kcal intake
3000 kcal output
No change in body weight
4000 kcal intake
2000 kcal output
Increase in body weight
2000 kcal intake
3000 kcal output
Decrease in body weight

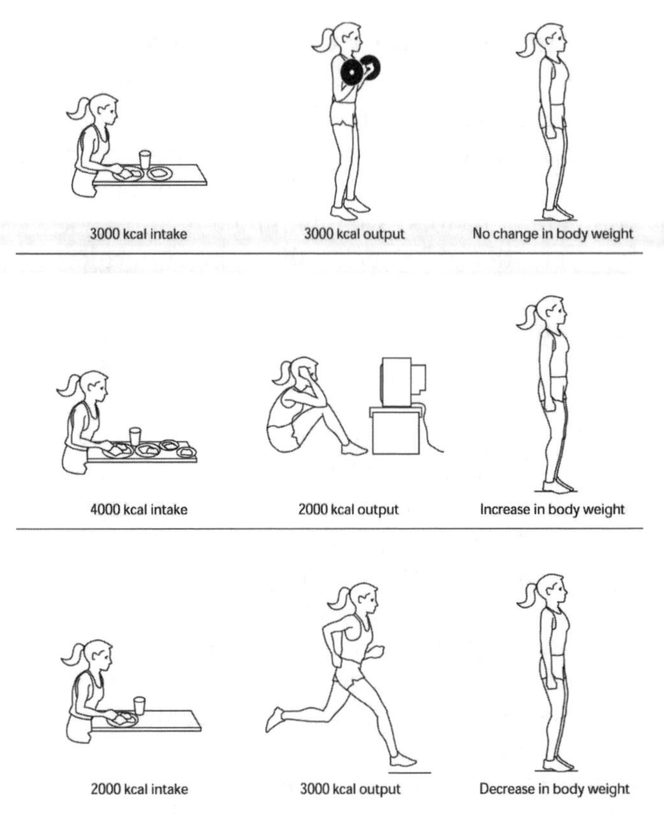

Figure 6.1: **Illustration of energy in versus energy out**

depend in part upon the methods used to create the energy imbalance. Diets that require drastic calorie reduction generally result in a substantial loss of fat and muscle tissue. In contrast, weight loss resulting from energy-burning exercise coupled with moderate calorie reduction results in a much greater proportion of fat loss.

Standards of Fatness

Average levels of body fatness associated with good health have been established for both women and men, but even these are subject to variation depending upon activity habits and interests. Adult non-athletic women should average 18 percent to 23 percent body fat while males should fall in the 12 percent to 15 percent range. As level of fatness increases so does the potential for health problems. When body fat exceeds 50 percent of a person's weight the condition may become life threatening. Table 6.2 illustrates average val-

TABLE 6.2: Standards of Fatness

Average Values for Body Fat
According to Age and Gender

Age	Men (%)	Women (%)
15	12.0	21.2
17	12.0	28.9
18-22	12.5	25.7
23-29	14.0	29.0
30-40	16.5	30.0
40-50	21.0	32.0

Adapted from Sharkey, 1997.

ues for body fat according to age and sex. Keep in mind that these are average values only, and do not necessarily represent the ideal.

Must We Get Fatter as We Get Older?

Although weight gain is generally considered a natural consequence of aging, there is actually no legitimate reason why you can't maintain the same level of fatness throughout life. The fact remains, however, that most women (and men) will get fatter (See Table 6.2) as they get older. This usually occurs due to one of the following scenarios ...

1. **Activity levels decline so energy requirements decrease.** Even though your eating habits may not have changed, you begin to add to your total fat mass. At about the same time you begin to lose muscle mass, on average about .5 pounds per year after the age of 30, so your metabolism slows and your energy requirements decrease even further. Because muscle is more dense than fat, your weight may not change significantly as muscle mass decreases and fat stores increase, but your body gradually takes on a softer, less defined shape.
2. **Body fat levels remain relatively constant but you gradually lose muscle mass.** This can occur with people who burn lots of calories through lower body aerobic exercise (running, cycling) but neglect to maintain upper body strength. Although their total amount of body fat remains about the

same, the relative percentage of body fat increases due to a gradual loss of muscle tissue.

Does Fatness Run in Families?

Children whose parents are obese are much more likely to be overweight than children whose parents are of normal weight. Whether fatness in the family is due to inherited factors or family lifestyle is a subject for debate. Studies of identical twins raised apart suggest that obesity has a genetic component. This is not surprising. We know that body shape, size, musculature and metabolism all have a genetic root, and each of those factors is indirectly linked to body weight and body composition. Does this mean we are at the mercy of our genes? Not necessarily. While it is true that individuals may differ in their predisposition for storing fat, the primary recipe for too much fat remains as it has always been — too many calories and/or too little exercise. Returning for a moment to the "fatness runs in families" argument, surveys indicate that families who are overweight tend to have pets that are overweight. No genetic link there!

Assessing Body Composition

Body fat measures can be obtained with a relatively high degree of accuracy. A few of the more common procedures are explained on the following pages.

Hydrostatic (Underwater) Weighing

Underwater weighing is based on the simple fact that "fat floats." Because fat is less dense than either bone or muscle, a woman with a greater percentage of fat for the same total body weight will weigh less in water. The subject is weighed without clothes and then submerged in water and weighed again. The difference between the person's scale weight and water weight, when corrected for the density of the water, equals the body's volume. This measure is further corrected to account for any air trapped in the body. Hydrostatic weighing provides the most accurate estimate of body composition but the procedure is not without limitations. For one, the amount air trapped in the lungs must be estimated. Individuals will also vary in bone density, and such variation is not accounted for. The underwater weighing procedure is usually more expensive and time consuming that alternative methods.

TABLE 6.3: Body Composition (% Body Fat) for Women					
	Age				
percentile	20-29	30-39	40-49	50-59	60+
99	<5.4	<7.3	<11.6	<11.6	<15.4
95	10.8	13.4	16.1	18.8	16.8
90	14.5	15.5	18.5	21.6	21.1
85	16.0	16.9	20.3	23.6	23.5
80	17.1	18.0	21.3	25.0	25.1
75	18.2	19.1	22.4	25.8	26.7
70	19.0	20.0	23.5	26.6	27.5
65	19.8	20.8	24.3	27.4	28.5
60	20.6	21.6	24.9	28.5	29.3
55	21.3	22.4	25.5	29.2	29.9
50	22.1	23.1	26.4	30.1	30.9
45	22.7	24.0	27.3	30.8	31.8
40	23.7	24.9	28.1	31.6	32.5
35	24.4	26.0	29.0	32.6	33.0
30	25.4	27.0	30.0	33.5	34.3
25	26.6	28.1	31.1	34.3	35.5

Adapted from the Insitute for Aerobics Research

Skin Fold Measurements

The skin fold technique centers around the relationship between the amount of fat located under the skin (subcutaneous fat) and the total amount of body fat. Skin fold measures are obtained at three body sites using a caliper. These values are then plugged into a formula to obtain a body fat estimate. An experienced tester can usually calculate percent body fat within an error range of 1 to 2 percent. Normative body composition data for women of various ages is provided in **Table 6.3.**

Body Mass Index

Body Mass Index (BMI) takes into account a person's height and weight to provide an estimate of body composition. To calculate BMI, perform the following steps ...

1. Divide your weight in pounds by 2.2 to convert to kilograms. This is your weight number.
2. Multiply your height in inches by 2.54 to convert to centimeters.

TABLE 6.4: Body Mass Index

The National Heart, Lung and Blood Institute's obesity standards say a person is overweight when his or her body mass index (BMI) is over 25–as measured by their weight in kilograms (one KG = 2.2 pounds) divided by their height in meters squared (one M = 3.3 feet). The following chart shows BMIs for some people. A BMI of 30 is considered obese.

					At risk for obesity					Obese	
(BMI)	21	22	23	24	25	26	27	28	29	30	31
Height	Weight										
5′0″	107	112	117	122	127	132	138	143	148	153	158
5′1″	111	117	122	127	132	138	144	148	154	159	164
5′3″	119	124	130	135	141	147	152	158	164	169	175
5′5″	126	132	138	144	150	156	162	168	174	180	186
5′7″	134	140	147	153	159	166	172	178	185	191	198
5′9″	142	149	155	162	169	176	182	189	196	203	209
5′11″	150	157	164	171	179	186	193	200	207	214	221
6′1″	158	166	174	181	189	196	204	211	219	226	234
6′3″	167	175	183	191	199	207	215	223	231	239	247

3. Divide your height in centimeters by 100 to convert to meters.
4. Take your height in meters and square it (multiply it by itself). This is your height number.
5. Divide your weight number by your height number to get your BMI.

If math isn't your strong point, you can also determine BMI through the use of a Body Mass Index Chart (Table 6.4).

The Panel on Energy, Obesity and Body Weight Standards uses the following table when classifying obesity according to BMI standards (See Table 6.5).

Bioelectric Impedance Analysis (BIA)

BIA is based on the assumption that the body's resistance to a small electric current passed through it is inversely related to the amount of muscle tissue contained within the body. In other words, the more muscle, the less resistance. Muscle has a greater water and electrolyte content that fat, and therefore is a better conductor of electricity. BIA is a simple procedure that takes only about five

TABLE 6.5

BMI	CLASSIFICATION
20-24	Desirable Range for Adult men and women
25-29.9	Grade 1 Obesity
30-40	Grade 2 Obesity
Greater than 40	Grade 3 Obesity (morbid obesity)

ACSM Guidelines

minutes to perform. It does have limitations, however. Body fat estimates obtained from BIA are less accurate and require more assumptions than estimates obtained from skin fold measurements. BIA also tends to overestimate body fat levels in very lean people and underestimate levels in obese individuals.

Body Fat Distribution

Your health may be affected not only by how much body fat you have, but also where the fat is located. Most people store body fat either around their middle (apple shape) or around their hips and buttocks (pear shape). Studies suggest that people with more abdominal fat are at increased risk of coronary artery disease, type II diabetes, high blood pressure and premature death, when compared to people who are equally fat but have more of the fat located in their hips and buttocks. The experts aren't exactly sure why this is so. It may be that fat stored in and around the abdomen is more likely to send free fatty acids directly to the liver where they can be used to synthesize cholesterol. Higher cholesterol levels can potentially increase the risk of heart disease.

A simple method used to estimate body fat distribution is the *Waist-to-Hip Ratio* (WHR). To determine WHR measure your waist size at the level of your navel and the circumference of your hips at the widest part of your buttocks. Record both measurements to the nearest quarter-inch. Divide the waist measurement by the hip measurement. For example, if you have a 28 inch waist and a hip circumference of 34 inches, your WHR is 0.82 . A ratio greater 0.86 for women (0.95 for men) places you at significantly greater risk for disease.

Muscular Fitness 7

When you speak of getting stronger, more toned and more shapely, you are really talking about improving muscular fitness. Muscular fitness has three primary components: strength, endurance and power. *Strength* is the maximum force that a muscle or muscle group can exert one time. A woman who can bench press 80 pounds has twice the strength of a woman who can bench press only 40 pounds. *Endurance* is a measure of a muscle or group of muscles ability to sustain repeated movements. The woman who can perform 20 push-ups has greater muscular endurance than a woman who can perform only 10 push-ups. *Power* is the explosive aspect of muscular fitness, expressed as a measure of how quickly strength can be displayed through a range of motion. Women competing in sports such as soccer, basketball and volleyball place a premium on the ability to produce explosive movement. For these individuals muscular power is more important than absolute strength.

All aspects of muscular fitness can be improved through resistance training. In addition to the obvious benefits of toning and strengthening your muscles, resistance training can improve balance, stimulate greater bone density and enhance coordination. Preserving muscle mass, particularly as we get older, plays a key role in maintaining normal body weight. Lean muscle is the engine that moves our body from one place to another. While a car engine runs on gasoline, our human engine is fueled by calories —roughly 30 to 50 calories per pound of muscle per day. The more muscle packed onto your frame the greater number of calories your body will burn every minute of every hour of every day.

The Training Overload

To improve muscular fitness you must move your muscles out of their normal comfort zone, a practice commonly referred to as *overloading* the muscle. Maximum strength gains are developed through a program of low repetitions coupled with heavy weight. Improvement is linked to muscle growth resulting from increases in contractile proteins and connective tissues. Muscle endurance is best developed through a program of higher repetitions and lesser weight. Improvements occur due to increased number of mitochondria, enhanced aerobic enzyme systems, and increased number of capillaries, adaptations that create more efficient aerobic pathways within the muscle fibers.

Resistance Training Programs

Isotonic training is based around changes in muscle length. *Concentric* contractions occur as the muscle shortens; *eccentric* contractions occur as the muscle lengthens. For example, when performing a bicep curl the concentric contraction occurs as you pull the dumbbell upward toward your shoulder. The eccentric contraction occurs as you lower the dumbbell to the original starting position. Free-weight training is the most popular method of isotonic training.

Isometric training involves pushing or pulling against an immovable object. Your muscles do not change in length during isometric exercise, so strength gains are not uniform throughout a range-of-motion. There is an element of risk associated with isometric contractions because they tend to elevate blood pressure. Although this will not usually pose a problem for a person whose blood pressure is within normal limits, it can be potentially dangerous for someone who suffers from hypertension.

Isokinetic training subjects the muscles to near maximal levels of resistance throughout an entire range of movement. Isokinetic

How Your Muscles Work

Muscle cells contain long strands of protein aligned next to one another. When you decide to move a specific body part, the brain sends a message to nerve cells to stimulate the muscles in that area. A chemical reaction then takes place in the muscle that causes the long strands of protein to slide toward and over one another, shortening the length of the muscle cells. For example, when you flex your bicep you are actually watching the muscle shorten and bulge upward as the protein strands slide over one another. Regular strength training causes the bundles of protein strands inside your muscles to grow larger. That is why your muscles look bigger and more defined.

Changes in Muscle Fiber

Skeletal muscle is composed of two different fiber types. *Fast twitch fibers* can generate a large amount of force but fatigue rather rapidly. *Slow twitch fibers* generate lesser amounts of force but can sustain the effort for a longer period of time. Research suggests that your muscles will selectively use a combination of fibers in response to the type of training. Explosive activities such as sprinting, jumping and weight lifting recruit a preponderance of fast twitch fibers. Endurance activities such as jogging, cycling and walking recruit a greater percentage of slow twitch fibers. Such findings suggest that we can selectively train the different types of muscle fiber, although to what extent is still unclear. High resistance/low-repetition (*muscular strength*) training involves a higher percentage of fast twitch fibers while lower resistance/higher repetition (*muscular endurance*) training utilizes a higher percentage of slow twitch fibers.

machine-based exercise stimulates the development of functional strength and is the preferred method of training for competitive athletes seeking a performance edge.

Gender Differences

Prior to puberty boys are not much stronger than girls. Afterward the strength differences get much greater and tend to persist throughout adult life. How much of the difference is due to physiological factors and how much to cultural factors remains unclear. It is well documented that higher levels of testosterone enable boys to develop bigger and stronger muscles than girls, although a portion of strength differences between the sexes may be due to the fact that men are culturally more motivated than women to lift weights and develop stronger muscles.

The Effects of Aging

Strength gradually declines after reaching a peak in the mid-twenties. The decrease can be attributed in large part to diminished *quantity* of muscle tissue rather than to *qualitative* changes within the muscle itself. In simple terms, that means we can slow the aging process by preserving muscle mass. Studies show that regu-

Setting the Limits

Genetics play a role in how tall you are, how heavy you are, and how strong you are. Each of us comes into the world with a certain percentage of slow twitch *(endurance)* and fast twitch *(strength)* muscle fiber. Those possessing a greater percentage of fast twitch fiber have a greater potential for strength development. Studies show that competitive women weight lifters have a greater percentage of fast twitch muscle fiber than non-lifters. How much of the difference is inherited and how much is due to a training effect remains unclear.

larly trained muscles can maintain levels of strength up to ages in the 70s.

How Strong are You?

Obtaining a reliable estimate of muscular strength and endurance is important for a number of reasons. It provides information useful for the development of appropriate resistance training programs. It provides a benchmark for the type of effort required to generate the training overload. It ensures that you do not initially place too much stress on muscles and connective tissues. It allows for the formation of believable and achievable training goals. Finally, it enables you to make future comparisons as you progress through the program.

Separate tests are used to assess upper body, lower body and general trunk strength. Table 7.1 lists three simple exercise tests that can provide an estimate *(low-medium-high)* of muscular strength and endurance.

TABLE 7.1

WOMEN

Exercise	Low	Medium	High	Estimate
Pull-up(reps)	20	20-30	30+*	Upper body strength
Push-up(reps)	10	10-20	30+	Upper body endurance
Sit-up (reps)	25	25-40	40+	Trunk endurance

Women perform a modified pull-up

Adapted from Sharkey, 1997.

TABLE 7.2: Estimating One-Repitition Maximum (Bench Press)

% of I-RM:	100.0	93.5	91.0	88.5	86.0	83.5	81.0	78.5	76.0	73.5
Reps:	1	2	3	4	5	6	7	8	9	10
Weight lifted (lbs).	0.0	0.0	0.0	0.0	0.0	0.0	0.0	0.0	0.0	0.0
	5.0	4.7	4.5	1.1	4.3	4.2	4.1	3.9	3.8	3.7
	10.0	9.4	9.1	8.9	8.6	8.4	8.2	7.9	7.6	7.4
	15.0	14.0	13.7	13.3	12.9	12.5	12.2	11.8	11.4	11.0
	20.0	18.7	18.2	17.7	17.2	16.7	16.2	15.7	15.2	14.7
	25.0	23.4	22.8	22.1	21.5	20.9	20.2	19.6	19.0	18.4
	30.0	28.1	27.3	26.6	25.8	25.0	24.3	23.6	22.8	22.1
	35.0	32.7	31.9	31.0	30.1	29.2	28.4	27.5	26.6	25.7
	40.0	37.4	36.4	35.4	34.4	33.4	32.4	31.4	30.4	29.4
	45.0	42.1	41.0	39.8	38.7	37.6	36.5	35.3	34.2	33.1
	50.0	46.8	45.5	44.3	43.0	41.8	40.5	39.3	38.0	36.8
	55.0	51.4	50.1	48.7	47.3	45.9	44.6	43.2	41.8	40.4
	60.0	56.1	54.6	53.1	51.6	50.1	48.6	47.1	45.6	44.1
	65.0	60.8	59.2	57.5	55.9	54.3	52.7	51.0	49.4	47.8
	70.0	65.5	63.7	62.0	60.2	58.5	56.7	55.0	53.2	51.5
	75.0	70.1	68.3	66.4	64.5	62.6	60.8	58.9	57.0	55.1
	80.0	74.8	72.8	70.8	68.8	66.8	64.8	62.8	60.8	58.8
	85.0	79.5	77.4	75.2	73.1	71.0	68.9	66.7	64.6	62.5
	90.0	84.2	81.9	79.7	77.4	75.2	72.9	70.7	68.4	66.2
	95.0	88.8	86.5	84.1	81.7	79.3	77.0	74.6	72.2	69.8
	100.0	93.5	91.0	88.5	86.0	83.5	81.0	78.5	76.0	73.5
	105.0	98.2	95.6	92.9	90.3	87.7	85.1	82.4	79.8	77.2
	110.0	102.9	100.1	97.4	94.6	91.9	89.1	86.4	83.6	80.9
	115.0	107.5	104.7	101.8	98.9	96.0	93.2	90.3	87.4	84.5
	120.0	112.2	109.2	106.2	103.2	100.2	97.2	94.2	91.2	88.2
	125.0	116.9	113.8	110.6	107.5	104.4	101.3	98.1	95.0	91.9
	130.0	121.6	118.3	115.1	111.8	108.6	105.3	102.1	98.8	95.6
	135.0	126.2	122.9	119.5	116.1	112.7	109.4	106.0	102.6	99.2
	140.0	130.9	127.4	123.9	120.4	116.9	113.4	109.9	106.4	102.9
	145.0	135.6	132.0	128.3	124.7	121.1	117.5	113.8	110.2	106.6
	155.0	140.3	136.5	132.8	129.0	125.3	121.5	117.8	114.0	110.3
	160.0	144.9	141.1	137.2	133.3	129.4	125.6	121.7	117.8	113.9
	165.0	149.6	145.6	141.6	137.6	133.6	133.7	125.6	121.6	117.6
	170.0	154.3	150.2	146.0	141.9	137.8	137.7	129.5	125.4	121.3
	175.0	159.0	154.7	150.5	146.2	142.0	141.8	133.5	129.2	125.0
	180.0	163.6	159.3	154.9	150.5	146.1	145.8	137.4	133.0	128.6

TABLE 7.3: Leg Strength

One Repetition Maximum Leg Press
Leg Press Weight Ratio = Weight Pushed/Body Weight

	Age					
Percentile	<20	20-29	30-39	40-49	50-59	60+
99	>1.88	>1.98	>1.68	>1.57	>1.43	>1.43
95	1.88	1.98	1.68	1.57	1.43	1.43
90	1.85	1.82	1.61	1.48	1.37	1.32
85	1.81	1.76	1.52	1.40	1.31	1.32
80	1.71	1.68	1.47	1.37	1.25	1.18
75	1.69	1.65	1.42	1.33	1.20	1.16
70	1.65	1.58	1.39	1.29	1.17	1.13
65	1.62	1.53	1.36	1.27	1.12	1.08
60	1.59	1.50	1.33	1.23	1.10	1.04
55	1.51	1.47	1.31	1.20	1.08	1.01
50	1.45	1.44	1.27	1.18	1.05	.99
45	1.42	1.40	1.24	1.15	1.02	.97
40	1.38	1.37	1.21	1.13	.99	.93
35	1.33	1.32	1.18	1.11	.97	.90
30	1.29	1.27	1.15	1.08	.95	.88
25	1.25	1.26	1.12	1.06	.92	.86

Adapted from the Insitute for Aerobics Research

You can use the *one-repetition maximum (1-RM) bench press test* to obtain a more definitive measure of upper body strength The test consists of lifting 50 to 75 percent of your body weight for a certain number of reps. Your 1-RM is calculated from the number of reps you complete. Determine your 1-RM from Table 7.2. A spotter must be present when conducting the test.

Muscular strength can also be expressed in terms *of the amount of weight you can push or pull compared to your body weight.* Relative measures actually provide a more representative estimate of strength than absolute measures, particularly for women because they are typically smaller than men. Tables 7.3 and 7.4 provide normative data for women on lower body strength (1-RM leg press) and upper body strength (1-RM bench press).

You can obtain an estimate of muscular endurance by performing the following simple tests.

TABLE 7.4: Upper Body Strength

One Repetition Maximum Bench Press
Bench Press Weight Ratio = Weight Pushed/Body Weight

	Age					
percentile	<20	20-29	30-39	40-49	50-59	60+
99	>.88	>1.01	>.82	>.77	>.68	>.72
95	.88	1.01	.82	.77	.68	.72
90	.83	.90	.76	.71	.61	.64
85	.81	.83	.72	.66	.57	.59
80	.77	.80	.70	.62	.55	.54
75	.76	.77	.65	.60	.53	.53
70	.74	.74	.63	.57	.52	.51
65	.70	.72	.62	.55	.50	.48
60	.65	.70	.60	.54	.48	.47
55	.64	.68	.58	.53	.47	.46
50	.63	.65	.57	.52	.46	.45
45	.60	.63	.55	.51	.45	.44
40	.58	.59	.53	.50	.44	.43
35	.57	.58	.52	.48	.43	.41
30	.56	.56	.51	.47	.42	.40
25	.55	.53	.49	.45	.41	.39

Adapted from the Insitute for Aerobics Research

✻ **Timed Sit-up Test.** Lie on your back with feet together and knees bent at 90 degrees. Interlock fingers behind your neck. Keep your heels in contact with the floor throughout the test. A partner should be present to hold your ankles firm. On the command, "Go" raise your upper body to the up position as shown in Figure 7.1. Immediately lower your body until the upper part of your shoulder blades contact the floor. Perform as many sit-ups in correct form as possible in 60 seconds.

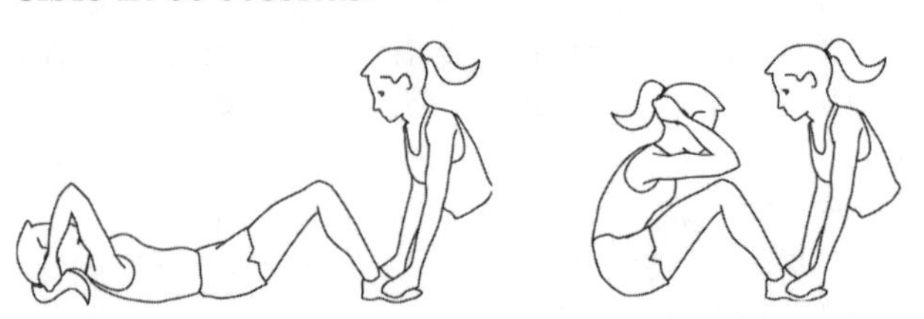

Figure 7.1: **Basic sit-up positions**

TABLE 7.5: Timed Sit-up Test

Women (reps per minute)

Age	40-49	50-59	60+
Excellent	29-38+	24-30+	17-28+
Good	24-28	20-23	11-16
Fair	20-23	14-19	6-10
Poor	14-19	10-13	3-5
Very Poor	13 or less	9 or less	2 or less

Performance norms for the 60-second sit-up test are listed in Table 7.5.

✳ **Modified Push Up Test**. Assume the *modified knee push-up* position with ankles crossed, knees bent at a 90-degree angle, back straight, hands shoulder-width apart, and head up. Lower your body until your chest touches the floor. Keep your back straight at all times. Perform each push-up to a straight arm position. The maximum number of push-ups

TABLE 7.6: Modified Push-Up Test

	Age				
Percentile	20-29	30-39	40-49	50-59	60+
99	>70	>56	>60	>31	>20
95	45	39	33	28	20
90	42	36	28	25	17
85	39	33	26	23	15
80	36	31	24	21	15
75	34	29	21	20	15
70	32	28	20	19	14
65	31	26	19	18	13
60	30	24	18	17	12
55	29	23	17	15	12
50	26	21	15	13	8
45	25	20	14	13	6
40	23	19	13	12	5
35	22	17	11	10	4
30	20	15	10	9	3
25	19	14	9	8	2

Adapted from ACSM Guidelines

performed consecutively without rest is your score. Performance norms for the modified push up test are provided in Table 7.6.

Aerobic Fitness 8

Aerobic fitness, also referred to as cardiovascular and cardio respiratory endurance, is a measure of the body's capacity to take in, transport and utilize oxygen. Your level of aerobic fitness is closely linked to the efficiency of the heart and circulatory system. A strong heart and healthy blood vessels ensure that stamina and energy levels remain high because your body is better equipped to supply the working muscles with oxygen. You feel younger, look younger, and from a physical point-of-view, are even able to act younger.

The term *aerobic* literally means in the presence of oxygen. During aerobic exercise you take in sufficient oxygen to meet the immediate needs of the active muscles. When exercise intensity goes beyond your ability to supply oxygen the body will automatically shift to *anaerobic* (without oxygen) energy pathways. Lactic acid, an energy transporter and by-product of high-intensity exercise, accumulates in the muscles during anaerobic activity. Excessive build-up of lactic acid interferes with muscle function and also causes feelings of fatigue and discomfort. For that reason it is not possible to exercise in an anaerobic state for an extended period of time.

The Oxygen Transport System

The cardiovascular and respiratory systems play important roles in the transport and delivery of oxygen to the muscles. Components of these systems related to oxygen transport are collectively referred to as the *oxygen transport system.* Regular aerobic exercise elicits changes in the oxygen transport system that enable it to function more efficiently. This in turn enables you to exercise harder and for longer periods before shifting into an anaerobic state. In performance terms, your capacity to perform physical work is increased. You've become more physically fit.

Sport scientists regard *VO_2 max*, defined as the highest rate of oxygen consumption attainable during maximal exercise, as the standard measure for aerobic fitness. VO_2 max is measured in mil-

> ### The Upper Limit?
>
> Cross-country skiing is considered by many to be the ultimate endurance exercise. Measured values for VO_2 max appear to support that contention. Values in excess of 80 ml/kg. min have been observed among elite male cross-country skiers. The highest VO_2 max ever recorded for a male was obtained from testing of a champion Norwegian cross-country skier who registered a value of 94 ml/kg. min. The highest recorded value for a female, obtained from testing of a Russian cross-country skier, is 77 ml/kg. min.

liliters per kilogram of body weight per minute (ml/kg.min). Active college-age women demonstrate average VO_2 max values of 38 to 42 ml/kg.min. College-age men average 44 to 50 ml/kg. min. Highly trained endurance athletes may post scores in excess of 60 ml/kg. min. Values for VO_2 max decrease an average of about 1 percent per year in sedentary adults.

Factors Affecting Aerobic Fitness

A number variables interact to determine your level of aerobic fitness at any given time, as well as your maximum attainable aerobic capacity. Some of these factors will respond positively to training; others do not.

Genetics. Of all the factors affecting our capacity for aerobic endurance, genetics may play the single most important role. It is estimated that inherited traits are responsible for as much as 50 percent of the total influence. The size of our heart, the capacity of our respiratory system, the density of red cells and hemoglobin, and the percentage of slow-twitch and fast-twitch muscle fiber are all genetically-linked traits. We also inherit mitochondria, the energy producing units of our muscles, from the maternal side of our family. The contention that world-class athletes are born with a decided advantage has been supported by longitudinal studies of elite endurance athletes who have stopped training but continue to maintain high VO_2 max values for many years afterward. Although measured levels of VO_2 max gradually decreased after years in a sedentary state, they remained extremely high when compared to general population norms.

Gender. Prior to puberty boys and girls demonstrate little difference in aerobic power. As girls get older they begin to lag behind. Clear cut gender differences become even more dramatic in adulthood. Young women, on average, demonstrate 15 percent to 25 percent less aerobic capacity than young men. A portion of the difference can be attributed to the fact that women, as a group, are not as physically active as men. Activity levels can't account for all of the difference, however. Even highly trained female endurance athletes score lower on measures of VO_2 max than men of similar age and training status. The variance may be due in part to the fact that men have higher concentrations of hemoglobin, the oxygen-carrying compound found in red blood cells, than do women. Women, on average, also have a greater percentage of body fat than men, are smaller in stature, and have less muscle mass, physical characteristics that tend to limit aerobic capacity. Despite these differences, women have made significant strides over the past couple of decades toward closing the performance gap with men. Dramatic improvements in events such as 10K and marathon runs clearly suggest that women can develop high levels of aerobic fitness if provided the same training opportunities as men.

Age. VO_2 max tends to decrease as we get older. Reasons for the drop off aren't always obvious. We know that most people gain weight as they age, and as body weight goes up the calculated VO_2

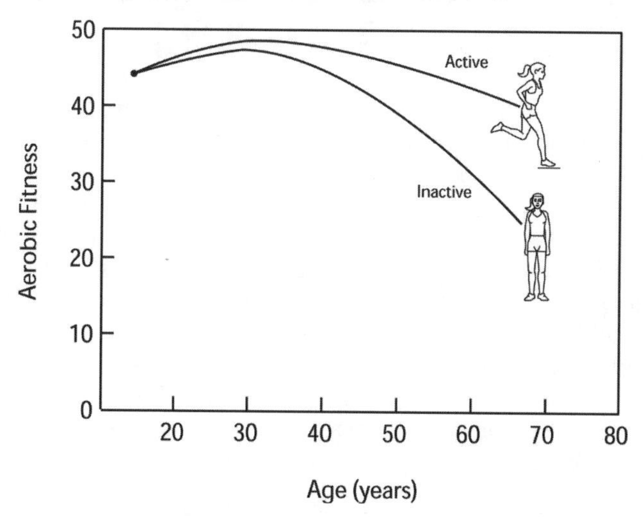

Figure 8:1: Age and aerobic fitness (VO_2 max).

max automatically goes down. Decreased activity levels also play a contributing role. Both body weight and activity levels are controllable factors, so a decline in aerobic fitness due either or both is not an inevitable consequence of aging. You can minimize the loss if you remain physically active and maintain normal weight.

Body Fat Levels. Because VO_2 max is calculated per unit of body weight (ml/kg. min.) your level of aerobic fitness will decline as you get heavier. This relationship provides a clear example of how the various parameters of physical fitness are intertwined, and how positively impacting one factor will in most cases positively influence another.

Training. Endurance exercise of sufficient duration, intensity and frequency will improve aerobic capacity by:

1. Increasing total blood volume and oxygen carrying capacity.
2. Producing a training effect in the slow-twitch muscle fibers specifically used for aerobic exercise.
3. Improving the muscles' ability to produce energy aerobically as metabolism shifts from carbohydrates to fat. From a health standpoint this is an important adaptation because it promotes fat loss, lowers blood fat levels, and in the process reduces your risk of cardiovascular disease.

VO_2 max Treadmill Test

The most accurate measure of aerobic fitness can be obtained by a laboratory test called the maximal oxygen uptake (VO_2 max) test. The procedure requires a treadmill and a metabolic measurement system to quantify oxygen, carbon dioxide, and the volume of expired air. The subject wears a mouthpiece to direct expired air into the analyzer. After a brief warmup she begins walking or running on the treadmill. Exercise intensity is increased incrementally every minute or so, and oxygen intake is computed every minute. The test ends when the subject can no longer keep pace with the treadmill, or when the measured oxygen intake levels off despite increasing exercise intensity. The test usually takes about 10 minutes to complete.

Note: *Subjects must undergo a health risk assessment and sign an informed consent form prior to testing.*

How Fit are You?

Maximal exercise tests provide the most accurate measure of aerobic power. Testing is usually conducted in a lab setting where VO_2 max is measured by direct analysis of expired gases. The procedure requires special equipment operated by trained personnel, and the testing protocol may be time consuming. The tests also present a substantial level of cardiovascular stress for the person being tested, so they may not be appropriate for older adults or individuals who have a history of heart and circulatory disease (See sidebar on preceding page: VO_2 max Treadmill Test).

Sub-maximal running and walking tests provide estimates of VO_2 max, or they rank performance according to national norms for gender and age. The tests are simple to administer and estimates of VO_2 max are relatively easy to compute. The objective is to cover the greatest distance possible in the time allotted, so your level of motivation at the time of testing will influence results. Running and walking tests have a slight degree of risk associated with them, so you should clear such testing with your physician.

* ***Cooper 12-Minute Test.*** Your goal is to cover as much ground as possible in 12 minutes. The distance covered (in miles) can be plugged into the following equation to obtain a reliable estimate of VO_2 max.

  VO_2 max (ml/kg.min) = 35.97 (miles covered in 12 minutes) - 11.3

  For example, if you covered 1.2 miles in 12 minutes your estimated VO_2 max would be:

  VO_2max (ml/kg.min) = 35.97 X (1.2 miles) - 11.3 = 31.9 ml/kg.min

  The Institute for Aerobics Research provides national performance norms for the Cooper Test based upon the distance covered and age range. Use Table 8.1 to measure your performance against women of similar age.

* ***1.5 Mile Walk/Run Test.*** Your goal is to cover the 1.5 mile course as fast as possible. Walking is permitted, but running is preferred. After completing the test you should cool down by walking slowly for a few minutes. Refer to Table 8.1 to rate your performance versus women of similar age.

TABLE 8.1: Aerobic Power Tests (Women)

	Age 20-29			Age 30-39		
percentile	VO_2 max (ml/kg/min)	12 Min. Run Distance (miles)	1.5 Mile Run (time)	VO_2 max (ml/kg/min)	12 Min. Run Distance (miles)	1.5 Mile Run (time)
99	>53.03	>1.78	>8:33	>48.73	>1.66	>10:05
95	46.75	1.61	10:47	43.87	1.53	11:49
90	44.15	1.54	11:43	40.98	1.45	12:51
85	42.42	1.49	12:20	40.26	1.43	13:06
80	40.98	1.45	12:51	38.57	1.38	13:43
75	39.53	1.41	13:22	37.37	1.35	14:08
70	38.09	1.37	13:53	36.65	1.33	14:24
65	37.37	1.35	14:08	35.44	1.29	14:50
60	36.65	1.33	14:24	34.60	1.27	15:08
55	36.14	1.31	14:35	33.85	1.26	15:20
50	35.20	1.29	14:55	33.76	1.25	15:26
45	34.48	1.27	15:10	32.41	1.22	15:47
40	33.76	1.25	15:26	32.31	1.21	15:57
35	32.72	1.22	15:48	31.09	1.17	16:23
30	32.31	1.21	15:57	30.51	1.16	16:35
25	30.94	1.17	16:26	29.93	1.13	16:58

	Age 40-49			Age 50-59		
percentile	VO_2 max (ml/kg/min)	12 Min. Run Distance (miles)	1.5 Mile Run (time)	VO_2 max (ml/kg/min)	12 Min. Run Distance (miles)	1.5 Mile Run (time)
99	>46.75	>1.61	>10:47	>42.04	>1.48	>12:28
95	40.98	1.45	12:51	36.81	1.33	14:20
90	39.53	1.41	13:22	35.20	1.29	14:55
85	37.49	1.35	14:06	33.59	1.24	15:29
80	36.28	1.32	14:31	32.31	1.21	15:57
75	35.11	1.29	14:57	39.90	1.20	16:05
70	33.76	1.25	15:16	30.87	1.17	16:27
65	33.04	1.23	15:41	29.76	1.14	16:51
60	32.31	1.21	15:57	29.43	1.13	16:58
55	31.59	1.19	16:12	28.70	1.11	17:14
50	30.87	1.17	16:27	28.22	1.10	17:24
45	30.58	1.16	16:34	27.98	1.09	17:29
40	29.45	1.13	16:58	26.85	1.06	17:55
35	29.43	1.12	16:59	26.13	1.04	18:09
30	28.25	1.10	17:24	25.48	1.02	18:23
25	27.98	1.09	17:29	25.09	1.01	18:31

Adapted from ACSM Guidelines for Exercise Testing and Prescription

TABLE 8.2: One Mile Walk Test

At a quarter-mile track (try the nearest high school), walk four times around carrying a stopwatch or a watch with a second hand to record your time. Go as briskly as you are able, then compare your time to the chart below to determine how aerobically fit you are.

Age	40-49	50-59	60-69	70-79
Excellent	<14:12	<14:42	<15:06	<18:18
Good	14:12–15:06	14:42–15:36	15:06–16:18	18:18–20:00
Average	15:06–16:06	15:36–17:00	16:18–17:30	20:00–21:48
Fair	16:06–17:30	17:00–18:05	17:30–19:12	21:48–24:06
Poor	17:30+	18:05+	19:12+	24:06+

Adapted from Physical Fitness Certification Manual (Cooper Institute for Aerobic Research)

✳ ***One Mile Walk Test.*** Walk four times around a quarter-mile track as briskly as you can. Record your time to the nearest second. Compare your time with Table 8.2 to obtain your level of aerobic fitness.

Flexibility 9

Flexibility has two component parts. *Static flexibility* deals with the range-of-motion (ROM) around a joint, but does not take into account the stiffness or looseness of the joint throughout the movement. *Dynamic flexibility* takes into account the resistance of a joint during movement, and in that respect is probably more applicable to our daily activity patterns. Staying loose and limber should be one of your primary fitness goals. Common movements such as walking, running and dancing become more difficult as range-of-motion decreases. Because muscles and connective tissues become less elastic with age, stretching becomes increasingly important as we get older.

Factors Affecting Flexibility

A number of variables interact to determine flexibility around a joint or series of joints. Some of these factors are malleable and can be improved through stretching exercises. Others are permanent in nature and impose fixed limits on the range-of-motion possible in certain areas of the body.

Joint Structure. Skeletal structure sets limits on flexibility in and around some joints. For example, the boney structure of your elbows determines the range-of-motion possible in that area. Short of surgery you can't do much about it. Ball-and-socket joints such as the hip and shoulder allow the greatest possible range-of-motion.

Age. Women and men alike become less flexible with age due in part to a process called fibrosis, where muscle fibers degenerate and are gradually replaced by a fibrous connective tissue. Fibrosis is an ongoing process and there is not much we can do to stop it.

Gender. Women tend to be more flexible than men across all age groups. Some of the difference is due to anatomical and physiological factors, although a substantial portion can be attributed to the nature and extent of activities routinely performed by men and women.

Connective Tissue. Flexibility in areas such as the ankle and hip is limited by soft tissues like tendons, ligaments, facial sheaths, joint capsules and even the skin. Stretching exercises can improve range-of-motion in these areas.

Activity Levels. Physically-active people tend to be more flexible than inactive people across all age groups. Ligaments and tendons become stiffer if they remain in a shortened (unstretched) position for extended periods of time. As the saying goes, if you don't use it you will lose it.

Frequency of Stretching. Range-of-motion will gradually decline if you fail to stretch on a regular basis. Perform stretching exercises at least every other day.

Types of Stretches

Ballistic and *static* stretches are the most common types of stretching exercises. Ballistic stretches extend the muscles to greater and greater lengths by using bouncing or bobbing motions. Static stretches employ a gradual and sustained extension of the target muscle. Static stretches are preferred because they do not elicit the stretch reflex (see sidebar). The likelihood of injury is also less because your muscles aren't subjected to sudden pressures and strains imposed by bouncing movements.

The Stretch Reflex

The human body contains a number of physiological checks and balances that prevent us from doing things, at least from a physical standpoint, that aren't in our best interests. Our built-in safeguard against over stretching is termed the *stretch reflex*. When the body senses that muscle fibers are stretching too far or too swiftly, a nerve reflex sends a signal to the muscle(s) being stretched to contract. In effect, the stretch reflex opposes your efforts to elongate the muscle. The mechanism is stimulated by sudden changes in muscle length, a condition that can result from the pressures and strains imposed by the bobbing-type movements used in ballistic stretching. The slow and steady extension characteristic of static stretch exercises inhibits firing of the stretch reflex, and thus enables the muscle to attain greater extension during the stretch.

Assessing Flexibility

A couple of simple at-home tests can provide an estimate of how well you measure up on the flexibility scale. You will need a partner to assist you.

Standard Sit-and-Reach Test

The sit-and-reach test provides a measure of lower back and hamstring flexibility. Poor flexibility in these areas coupled with weak abdominal muscles has been identified as a primary cause of lower back pain in adults. You will need a 12-inch high box to administer the test.

Tape a yardstick on top of the box so that it extends 15" in front of the box. Sit with your bare feet up against the box, no more than 10 inches apart. Place one hand over the other with toes pointing up. Bend forward at the waist and, with both hands, try to touch your toes or reach beyond. Breathe normally during the test. Keep your hands together — do not lead with one hand. You can overlap your fingertips if you like, but you should keep them in contact with the yardstick or measuring portion of the sit-and-reach box. Hold the full stretch position for several seconds. The ability to touch your toes, or a least come close, is considered adequate flex-

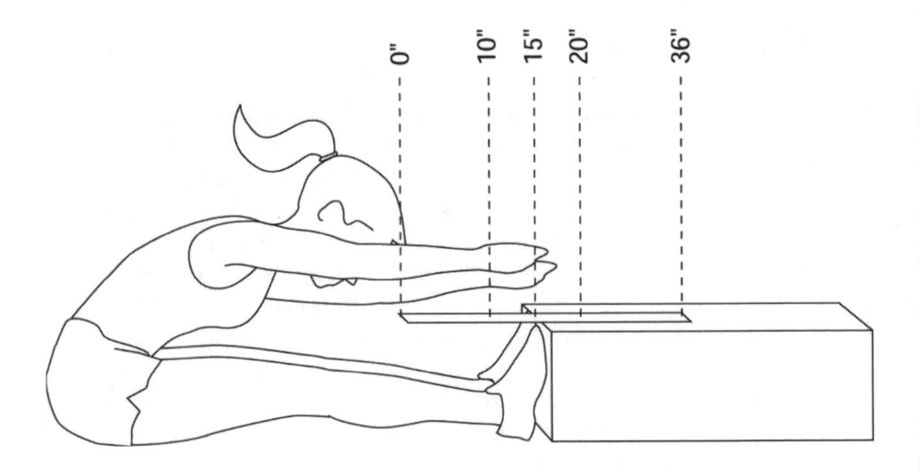

Figure 9.1: **Sit-and-reach test**

TABLE 9.1: Flexibility in Women
Sit-and-Reach (inches)

Age	*40-49*	*50-59*	*60+*
Excellent	20.5–22.8+	20.23–23+	19–23+
Good	19–20.4	18.5–20.2	17–18.9
Fair	17.3–18.9	16.8–18.4	15.5–16.9
Poor	15–17.2	14.8–16.7	13–15.4
Very Poor	14.9 or less	14.7 or less	12.9 or less

Adapted from ACSM Guidelines

ibility (See Figure 9.1). Your score is the most distant point reached on the yardstick (in inches). Take the best of three trials. The normative data provided in Table 9.1 provides an estimate of how you measure up in comparison to women in your age group.

Modified Sit-and-Reach Test (partner assisted)

The standard sit-and-reach test fails to take into account individual differences in arm and leg length, factors that can influence how far you can extend your arms and hands in relation to your feet. A modified version of the sit-and-reach test can be used to eliminate the effects of differing arm and leg length. Sit on the floor with your buttocks, shoulders and head in contact with the wall. Extend your legs with knees straight, and place the soles of

TABLE 9.2: Percentile Scores for the
Modified Sit-and-Reach Test

Percentile Rank	< 35 years	36–49 years	> 50 years
99	19.8	19.8	17.2
95	18.7	19.2	15.7
90	17.9	17.4	15.0
80	16.7	16.2	14.2
70	16.2	15.2	13.6
60	15.8	14.5	12.3
50	14.8	13.5	11.1
40	14.5	12.8	10.1
30	13.7	12.2	9.2
20	12.6	11.0	8.3

Adapted from Morton Publishing Co., 1987

your feet against a 12-inch high box. Position one hand on top of the other. Have your partner position a yardstick on top of the box with the zero end nearest to you. Reach forward as far as possible without allowing your head and shoulders to come away from the wall. Your partner repositions the yardstick so that the zero end touches your outstretched fingers. The yardstick must remain in this position until the test is completed. Continue to lean forward slowly, allowing your head and shoulders to move away from the wall, and slide your fingers forward along the top of the yardstick. Make three slow, forward movements. On the third lean forward as far as possible and hold this position for at least 2 seconds. Your partner records how far your fingers have moved forward along the yardstick. Two separate trials are taken. The mean of the two trials is recorded as your sit-and-reach score. You can get a rough idea of your percentile rank for the test by comparing your score to those provided in Table 9.2.

Section III
Becoming Fit: The Process

Knowledge is not enough, we must apply.
Willing is not enough, we must do.

– Goethe

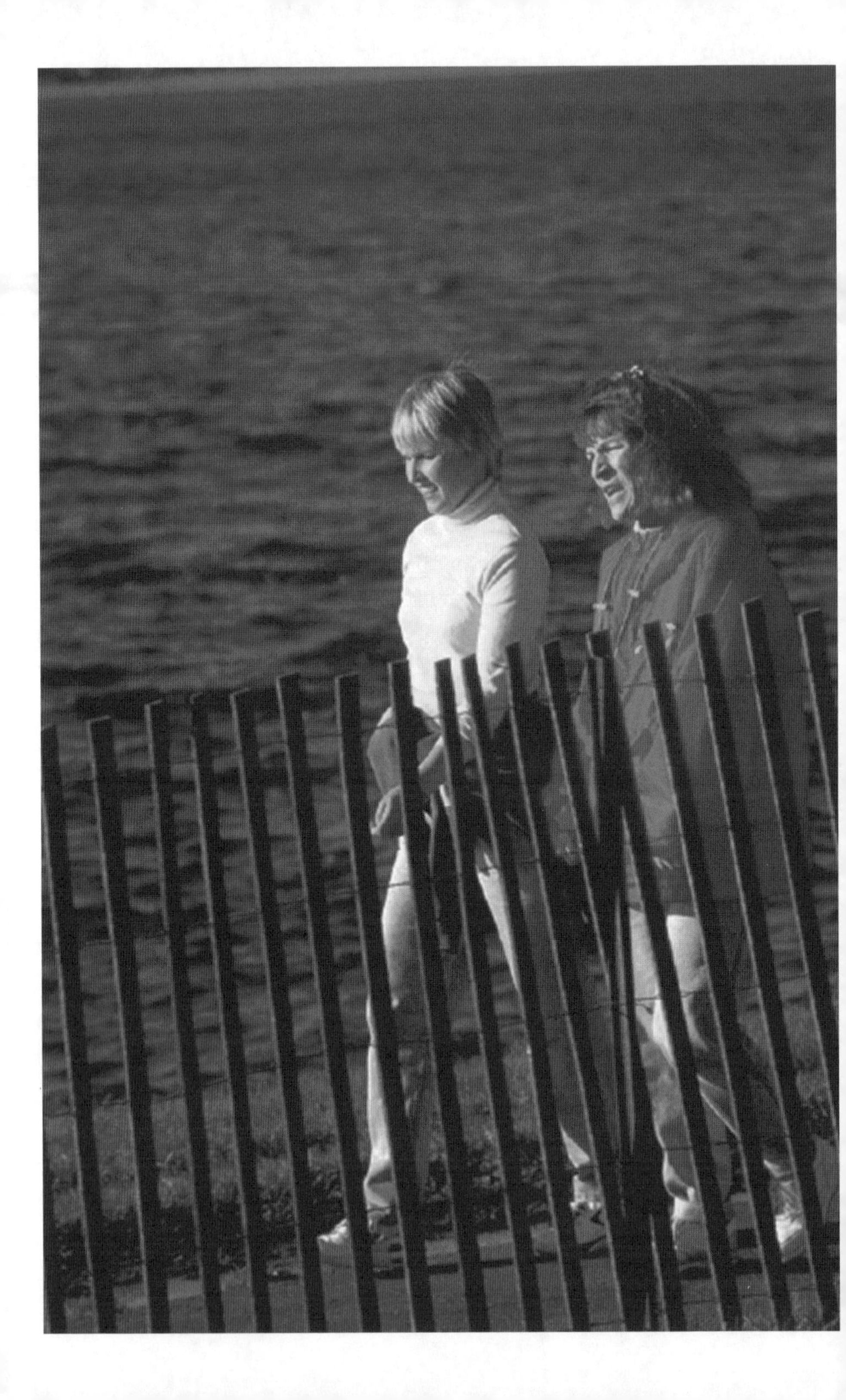

Planning for Success 10

Have you ever entered a race that did not have a clearly defined course or finish line? Probably not. I would find it very difficult to stay motivated if I did not know which way to go or where the road might lead. Surprisingly, many people approach the process of becoming fit in just that manner. They enter the race knowing they want to get stronger, leaner, trimmer and toned, but have no clear idea of how to do it. They end up expending a great deal of energy and effort, fail to see tangible results, gradually lose their enthusiasm and ultimately drop out of the race.

Transforming dreams into reality will not occur by chance. There must be method to your madness! Dreams are merely a starting point. They provide us with a vision of the big picture, of where we hope to be one, five or ten years down the road. Dreams stretch our imagination and identify the finish line, but they don't tell us how to get there. That is where our goals come into play. Goals define the day-to-day behaviors required to transform dreams into reality. Goals chart the course, provide benchmarks to measure progress, and provide an opportunity to experience daily successes. Whether your dream is to accumulate a large nest egg for retirement, lose the spare tire around your middle or complete that novel you've been threatening to write for the past decade, the importance of making daily progress toward your goals cannot be overstated. The cumulative effects of small successes experienced daily can be staggering over the long term.

Effective Goal-Setting

You definitely won't hit a target if you don't have one. It is imperative that you clearly identify your finish line and chart out a series of steps that will ultimately lead you there. Consider the following guidelines when formulating your fitness goals.

1. **Write It Down.** Put your goal statements on paper. Written goals become a legitimate contract — with yourself. Post the contract where you will see it every day.

2. **Be Positive.** State specifically what you will do as opposed to what you won't do. For example, the goal statement *I will never eat cake again* can be better rephrased to say *I will limit fat calories to 25 percent of my total calorie intake every day.* That statement takes a more positive approach to the situation, and also allows more flexibility in food choices.
3. **Be Precise.** Define your targets a clearly as possible. The more precise your goals, the easier it will be to focus your efforts and monitor progress. The goal statement *I will perform 3 sets of 30 push-ups every day* is much more precise than *I will do push-ups every day.*
4. **Prioritize.** Decide which aspects of becoming fit are most important to you and prioritize accordingly. Do you want to lose weight? Add muscle? Reshape your body? Prioritizing will enable you to effectively channel your efforts to produce maximum results in the shortest period of time.
5. **Be Specific.** Set specific, measurable, short- and long-term goals. The statement *I want to get in better shape* is a general desire, not a specific goal. *I will exercise a minimum of five days a week for 30 minutes or more each day* is a more specific, measurable short-term goal. *I will reduce my level of body fat to 20 percent* is a specific, measurable, long-term goal. Setting specific short- and long-term goals will focus your efforts and also provide a means for evaluating progress. If you consistently find yourself falling short, then you can figure out the reasons why and take appropriate action.
6. **Be Realistic**. While it is important to establish goals that stretch your physical and mental limits, it is equally important that your goals be realistic and attainable. Unrealistic expectations will eventually lead to frustration and exercise dropout. *I will lose 10 pounds of fat in one week* sounds like a great goal, but from a physiological standpoint it's just not possible.
7. **Set Performance Goals.** Focus on performance rather than outcomes. Performance goals spell out what you will do, not necessarily what you will accomplish by doing them. The goal statement *I will walk two miles every day* is a performance goal totally within your control. If you commit to do it, then you can do it. The goal statement *I will drop three*

dress sizes by my high school reunion next month is an outcome goal. Goals based purely on outcomes are more vulnerable to failure because of circumstances beyond your control.

8. **Set Action Goals.** Creating a "wish list" is not a legitimate substitute for goal-setting. The dream of completing a marathon is nothing more than a wish unless you take positive steps toward realization of that dream. Goal-directed behaviors that eventually prepare you to run a marathon will turn your dream into reality. Your goals should motivate you to take action each and every day. View the completion of each goal as one small step taking you closer to your ultimate objective.
9. **Seek Control.** Measure progress and overall level of accomplishment against your own standards and personal expectations. Compete with yourself rather than with others.
10. **Monitor Progress.** Achievement of short-term goals provides an on-going measure of progress toward the realization of your long-term goals. Chart your workouts and make note of any changes to your program. Keep a record of when you increase the resistance and by how much. Record the time and/or mileage covered when walking, running or biking each day. If there comes a point when you begin to question the effectiveness of your program, you will be able to look back and compare where you were then to where you are now.
11. **Evaluate and Adjust.** Periodically take a step back to assess your progress. You may find that your goal statements aren't challenging enough, that you are capable of doing more. On the other hand, if you are having difficulty sticking with your program, it is possible that you've set the bar too high. Becoming fit is a lifelong process, and change is an essential part of life. Be willing to make adjustments when necessary.

Experience Success Daily

From a fitness point-of-view, you are going to arrive somewhere down the road five, ten and twenty years from now. The real question is not whether you are going to reach that point in your life, but rather how you will look and feel once you get there.

By setting realistic short- and long-term fitness goals you will establish patterns of behavior that will shape your physical future. I can't stress enough the importance of doing something every day, however slight it may be, toward the realization of your fitness goals. The overall effects of your daily behaviors are cumulative. What you do today, tomorrow and the next day will play a role in how you look and feel two months from now. Granted, it won't have much of an effect if those are the only three days that you exercise during the next eight weeks. But if you program yourself to do something physical every day, or most every day, you will set into motion a process that can generate massive physical change over the long haul. Start slowly and experience success daily. As you begin to see tangible results you will become motivated to reach for even greater heights.

Weight Loss Basics 11

It's somewhat ironic that body fat, so easy to put on, seems so difficult to take off. Dieting has become a way of life for millions of women. In the quest for a thinner, more sexy body they bounce from one plan to the next with little success. Most lose weight initially, but the vast majority (over 90 percent) gain it back. Failure to keep the weight off has little to do with a lack of effort or willpower. It has everything to do with the fact that *diets just don't work!* The statistics don't lie. You will not lose weight and keep it off through dieting alone. It just can't be done. That being said, I can assure you that you already possess the power to lose fat permanently and reshape your body in the process. The key to unleashing that power is knowledge.

You May Be Surprised to Know That...

Not All Fat is Bad. The phrase "you can never be too rich or too thin" should not be taken literally. Your body requires a minimum level of fat, referred to as *essential fat*, to function normally. Essential fat comprises parts of our spinal cord, brain, nerves and cell membranes. It also serves as a cushion for internal organs and provides a layer of insulation against the cold. Essential fat comprises about 12 percent of a woman's body weight. A large portion is stored in the thighs, hips and breasts where it is readily available to nourish a baby during pregnancy. Higher levels of essential fat in women (men average 4%) is nature's way of telling us that a well-nourished baby is a healthy baby.

Calories Do Count. In today's high tech era of low-fat, reduced-fat, and no-fat foods, slick marketing has fostered an erroneous belief that all you need to do to lose weight is eliminate dietary fat. While consuming too much fat is a legitimate cause of weight gain, the fact remains that the mix of calories (fat, carbohydrate, protein) is of less consequence than the total number of calories you eat. Fat-free foods do not equate to calorie-free foods. Some fat-free products contain as many if not more calories than the foods they are designed to replace. The source of calories has merely been switched from fat to an increased sugar and starch content.

Your Body Has a Vote in Weight Loss. It has been theorized that humans have an internally programmed, predetermined level of fat that the body strives to maintain. Referred to as our *setpoint*, it is the amount of fat the body would carry naturally if we didn't worry about watching our weight. Conflicts arise when the body's natural setpoint does not coincide with our concept of ideal weight. For example, let's assume that you have set a personal goal of achieving 18% body fat but your setpoint has been programed to center around 23% fat. As fat levels dip below the setpoint your body senses something is amiss, and resists further weight loss by making internal adjustments to conserve fat. One way it does this is by depressing resting metabolic rate. Through no fault of your own, your body begins to burn fewer calories so the rate of weight loss slows or in some cases stops entirely.

You Can't Lose 30 Pounds in 30 Days. When it sounds to good to be true it usually is. If even one of these "effortless" weight loss gimmicks actually worked, millions of women would use it, stick with it, and thereby eliminate their lifelong struggle with too much body fat. That hasn't happened and in all likelihood won't.

A Little Goes A Long Way. If you are greatly overweight you don't have to lose huge amounts of weight to reap a number of positive health benefits. According to the American Heart Association a weight loss of only 5 percent will produce improvements in how well your heart pumps blood and also will also reduce the risk of sleep apnea, a breathing disorder characterized by hundreds of brief interruptions from sleep during the night. A 10 percent weight loss can significantly improve a person's blood profile, especially triglycerides and levels of the good HDL cholesterol.

Can You Alter Your Setpoint ?

Yes — but not by dieting! Exercise appears to be the key to adjusting our internal weight control mechanism. Studies demonstrate that food (calorie) intake usually decreases for sedentary overweight women and men who begin a program of regular exercise. When these people maintain an active lifestyle their calorie intake eventually achieves a balance with daily energy requirements, and their body weight stabilizes at a lower level. In effect, they've lowered their setpoint.

Understanding the Energy Equation

If you can put social, psychological and emotional factors aside — and that is no easy task — altering body weight is purely a matter of energy imbalance. Take in more calories than needed to fuel normal body functions and daily physical activity, and you will gain weight. Burn more calories than you consume, and you will lose weight. From a mathematical point-of-view that's all there is to it!

The *energy equation* provides a simple and straightforward explanation of how body fat levels fluctuate in response to the number of calories consumed compared with the number of calories burned. The equation can take three forms:

- ✳ Caloric intake <u>*equals*</u> calorie output — *body weight remains constant*
- ✳ Caloric intake <u>*exceeds*</u> calorie output — *body weight increases*
- ✳ Caloric intake <u>*less than*</u> calorie output — *body weight decreases.*

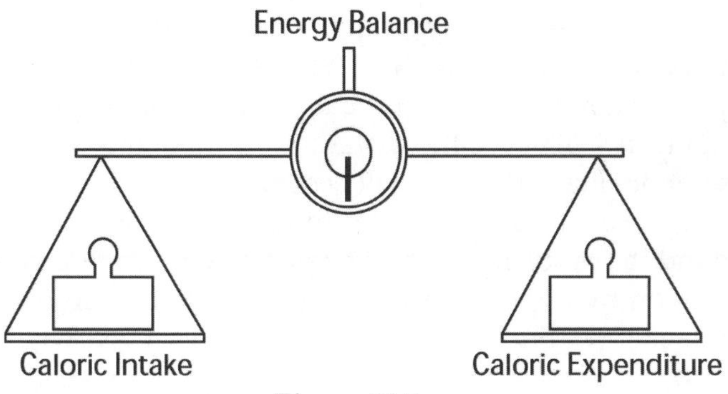

Figure 11.1

Manipulating the Energy Equation

There are two primary ways that you can manipulate the energy equation to work in your favor, and in doing so control your weight. You can either reduce the number of calories you consume or increase the number of calories you burn, or both.

Method #1: Consume Fewer Calories

Cutting calories is the method of choice for most people. Simple arithmetic would indicate that reducing calorie intake should auto-

What is a Calorie?

The calorie *(kilocalorie)* is a unit of energy, specifically defined as the amount of heat required to raise the temperature of 1 kilogram of water 1 degree Celsius. We obtain calories from the proteins, fats and carbohydrates contained in the foods we eat and drink. The number of calories burned during physical activity is influenced by several factors. In general, a larger person burns more calories at a given exercise intensity than will a smaller person.

matically result in weight loss. In the real world it's not that straightforward. We've discussed how nine of 10 people who attempt to lose weight by dieting alone (unsupplemented with exercise) regain the weight within the first year or two. The low success rate can be attributed to the fact that most dieters make a couple of fundamental assumptions that, if violated, limit the effectiveness of their diet.

Assumption #1: Energy expenditure will remain constant throughout the period of dieting. You can't count on this to occur. A very low calorie diet will gradually deplete carbohydrate stores, which in turn will cause the dieter to feel tired and lethargic. This makes it more likely that she will become less active, and as a result her energy expenditure decreases during the period of dieting. To compound the problem, her body responds to the perceived threat of starvation by depressing its resting metabolism in an effort to conserve energy. She requires fewer calories, even when at rest. Added to this is the fact that, as she begins to lose weight, the energy cost of moving a smaller body is reduced proportionately. The combined effect of all these changes is that her body burns fewer calories than before she started the diet, which makes it increasingly more difficult to lose weight.

Assumption #2: You will be able to stay on a diet until reaching your goal weight. There are several factors working against you here. Most diet plans place limits on the types and amounts of foods permitted, so it's understandable how a dieter can become frustrated and bored when required to eat the same types of foods in the same amounts at the same time of day. Social, cultural and environmental influences also take a toll. Virtually everywhere you go in our society there is food for the taking. Even the most strong-willed individuals must eventually come to grips with the question of whether they want to remain on a restrictive food plan for a lifetime.

Method #2: Burn More Calories

The only surefire way to increase energy expenditure is to become more active. Regular exercise can increase the number of calories burned in several ways. Aerobic exercise burns calories by raising metabolic rate over the *short term*. The longer and more intense the workout, the more calories you will burn. If the exercise is fairly vigorous your metabolic rate may remain elevated for an hour or more after the workout has ended. This "after-burn effect" enables your body to burn additional calories even after you've showered and left the gym. Strength-training plays an important role in *long term* weight maintenance. Every pound of lean muscle burns 30 to 50 calories a day. By maintaining muscle mass you will keep your metabolism elevated, and thereby increase the number of calories your body burns every minute of every hour of every day.

Studies demonstrate conclusively that exercise *must* play a role in achieving permanent weight loss. Due to a combination of myth and misinformation, this fact has been lost on many people. Let's take a few moments to dispel two of the most common myths concerning exercise and weight loss.

Myth #1: The more I exercise the more I'll eat – so why exercise? This belief is based upon the misconception that appetite will automatically increase in direct proportion to increased amounts of physical activity. The opposite usually takes place. Sedentary individuals who begin an exercise program often experience a decrease in appetite with up to one hour of daily, low level physical activity. In reality, regular exercise helps to control appetite rather than increase it.

Myth #2: It takes an inordinate amount of exercise to lose one pound of fat – so why exercise? This appears to be a valid argument. It is true that to lose one pound of body fat you must burn approximately 3500 calories above and beyond what you consume. That translates into a heck of a lot of exercise — jogging 30 miles, biking for 7 hours, skipping rope for 6 hours or a brisk 8 hour walk! On face value one might come to the conclusion that the

What Type of Exercise is Best?

Consistency and duration of exercise are more important than intensity when it comes to weight loss. It doesn't require intense workouts to fuel your fat-burning furnaces. For many people lower-intensity exercise actually pays higher dividends because it is more easily sustained. It requires less effort to walk 2 miles than it does to jog that distance. In both cases you will burn a similar number of calories; it merely takes you longer to do so when walking. The best type of exercise for weight loss is the one that you enjoy and will perform on a consistent basis.

potential return isn't worth the investment. If approached from a different perspective you can gain a greater appreciation for the important role exercise can play in achieving and maintaining your goal weight. The important point to be made is this — *the calorie burning effects of exercise are cumulative.* Take a brisk 20-minute walk each day for the next 30 days and the total energy expenditure will be roughly the same as running a marathon. In both cases you've burned about one pound of body fat. The only difference between the two is the rate of fat loss. Make that 20-minute walk a daily ritual (habit) and you will lose 10 pounds of fat by this time next year — and tone your legs in the process. (See sidebar — What Type of Exercise is Best?)

Weight Control Wisdom

You've no doubt figured it out by now that neither diet or exercise alone will do the job. Both options considered in and of themselves have obvious limitations. When taken together, however, they can provide a formidable weapon against the middle age spread. Simply cutting back on fat intake can reduce significantly the number of calories you consume. Most health experts recommend that no more than 30% of total calories come in the form of fat. At the same time you can use exercise to rev up your calorie-burning furnaces and speed the weight loss process. Formal exercise such as biking, jogging and stair climbing is great, but so are everyday activities such as walking, gardening and yard work. Whatever your choice of activity, it is essential to get your body moving on a regular basis. You can win your personal battle of the bulge by combining a healthy eating plan with regular calorie-burning exercise. The two-pronged fat attack provides the most flexibility and offers the greatest opportunity for long term success. It's really the only way to do it.

Can You Spot Reduce?

A variety of machines have been marketed claiming to stimulate fat loss in specific areas of the body. None have proven to work effectively. Heat belts, for example, have been promoted as a means to melt away the spare tire around your middle. In reality, they serve only to dehydrate and shrink body cells. Granted, if you measure your waistline immediately after wearing a heat belt, it may indeed be smaller — but only for a short while. Usually about the length of time it takes to gulp down a couple of large glasses of water. There is no known technology short of liposuction that will remove fat from specific areas of the body. Spot reduction of fat just doesn't work, although spot toning of muscle does.

12

7 Steps to Permanent Fat Loss

Step #1: Accept the Fact that You Become What You Eat!

A healthy low-fat diet is an essential part of every successful weight loss program. Exercise alone won't do it. You can run five miles a day and lift weights until you are blue in the face, but you won't lose the soft cushion around your middle if your diet is centered around creme-filled donuts and pie á là mode! What you eat on a daily, weekly and monthly basis will significantly impact your body weight as well as your ability to exercise on a regular basis. By eating the right foods in the right amounts, you can lose fat and at the same time maximize the energy reserves required to fuel daily workouts. Despite claims to the contrary, there are no magical foods that when taken in combination will speed fat loss. It is purely a matter of energy-in versus energy-out.

Nutrition Facts
Serving Size 4 pieces (50g)
Servings Per Container 5

Amount Per Serving

Calories 190	Calories from Fat 70
	% Daily Value*
Total Fat 8g	**13%**
Saturated Fat 1.5g	**8%**
Cholesterol 30mg	**10%**
Sodium 180mg	**8%**
Total Carbohydrate 26g	**9%**
Dietary Fiber 1g	**2%**
Sugars 16g	
Protein 2g	
Vitamin A 2% • Vitamin C 0%	
Calcium 2% • Iron 0%	

* Percent Daily Values are based on a 2,000 calorie diet. Your daily values may be higher or lower depending on your calorie needs:

		Calories: 2,000	2,500
Total Fat	Less than	65g	80g
Sat Fat	Less than	20g	25g
Cholesterol	Less than	300mg	300mg
Sodium	Less than	2,400mg	2,400mg
Total Carbohydrate		300g	375g
Dietary Fiber		25g	30g

* *ACTION STEP: Count Calories.* Most people have no idea how many calories they actually consume. Record everything that you eat and drink over the period of seven consecutive days. Try to eat normally during that time. Be meticulous and honest with your recordings.
* *ACTION STEP: Read Nutrition Labels.* Make smart food choices. Look for the heading **Nutrition Facts** on the package and pay particular attention to the following features...
  - *Standard Serving Size*: This information will enable you to compare the labeled serving size with the amount you normally eat, which is usually more but may be less than the listed serving size.

- *Percent Daily Value*: Provides information on the amount (percent) of certain nutrients contained in one serving.
- *Daily Values*: Provides reference values set by the government for sample 2,000- and 2500-calorie-a-day diets. Your needs may be greater or less than that listed on the label.

Be A Savvy Supermarket Shopper

1. ***Establish nutritional goals.*** Your diet should derive no more than 30 percent of calories from fat, of which 10 percent or less should be of the saturated, artery-clogging variety. Sixty to 65% of calories should come from carbohydrates, primarily complex carbohydrates, and the remainder from protein. Cholesterol and sodium intake should not exceed 300 and 2400 milligrams per day, respectively.
2. ***Make a shopping list***. The more thought you put into food selections and meal planning, the less likely that you will make poor choices.
3. ***Don't shop on an empty stomach***. Avoid impulse buying. Those creamy deserts and candy bars located at the checkout counter are even more enticing when you are hungry.
4. ***Study the store layout.*** Marketing experts plan store layouts so that you spend most of your money on items the store wants you to buy. Did you ever wonder why dairy products, meat, poultry, and seafood are located a good distance from the entrance to the store? This is not by coincidence. Almost everybody buys milk and meat products. To get to these items you must walk through the store, often along the perimeter where the bakery and deli are usually located. It's hard to resist the urge to "binge buy." All the more reason to have a plan and stick to it.
5. ***Be aware of nutritional loopholes***! Some foods are exempt from the nutritional labeling requirement. Milk is one such item. You would expect "low-fat" 2% milk to contain only 3 grams of fat per serving (8-ounce glass). It actually contains 5 grams of fat, of which 3 grams are saturated. This is not meant to imply that 2% milk is an unhealthy food, because it is not. Just a reminder that you can't believe everything you read unless, of course, you read it here!

TABLE 12.1: Determining Goal Weight

Present Weight:	140 pounds
% Body Fat:	30%
Fat Weight:	140 lbs X 0.30 = 42 pounds
Fat-free Weight:	140 lbs – 42 lbs. fat weight = 98 pounds
Goal (% fat):	20% (80% fat-free weight)
Goal Weight:	98 pounds/.80 = 122.5 pounds
Weight Loss Goal :	Present Weight - Goal Weight = **17. 5 pounds**

* *ACTION STEP: Learn the language.* Nutritional claims can be misleading if you aren't familiar with the terminology. Legal definitions of nutritional claims are listed below:
  - *Free:* The product contains a negligible amount of specific nutrient
  - *Reduced*: The food has at least a 25% reduction in nutrient compared to the regular product. *Note:* The claims "free" and "reduced" are often used in conjunction with the terms calorie, fat, cholesterol, saturated fat, sodium, and sugar.
  - *Low:* The food contains a small amount of a particular nutrient. The standards for various nutrients are:

    Low Fat – 3 grams or less fat per serving

    Low in Saturated Fat – 1 gram or less saturated fat per serving

    Low Cholesterol — 20 milligrams or less cholesterol per serving and 2 grams or less saturated fat per serving

    Low Sodium — 140 milligrams or less sodium per serving

    Low Calorie — 40 calories or less per serving.
  - *Lite or Light:* The product has one-third fewer calories than a comparable product, or 50 percent or less of the fat found in a comparable product.

Step #2: Determine Goal Weight

Ideal body weight is not necessarily the lowest possible level of body fat that you can achieve. In the absence of heart disease and related circulatory problems, there appears to be little health difference between the extremes of 12 percent and 30 percent body fat for women. Your target body weight should place you somewhere between those extremes.

✳ *ACTION STEP: Determine Target Body Weight.* Use the following calculations to obtain an estimate of your goal weight. The first provides a normal weight range (in pounds) for a person of your height. The second determines what you should weigh at a predetermined level of body fat.

Option #1. Although body composition analysis is the most accurate and reliable method of determining how much you should weigh, there is a simpler albeit less accurate method used to estimate the midpoint of a healthy weight range. The predicted value has a range of plus or minus 10 percent depending upon whether you have a small or large frame. To obtain your target weight, estimate 100 pounds for the first 5 feet of height. Add 5 pounds per inch thereafter.

Example: A woman who is 5 feet, 5 inches tall should weigh 100 lbs + 25lbs = 125 pounds plus or minus 10% (Weight range is 112.5 to 137.5 pounds).

Option #2. To use this procedure you must know your present level (percent) of body fat and body weight (lbs). Use the following formula to determine goal weight based on your desired level of body fat.

Goal Weight = lean body weight/1.00 - %fat desired

Table 12.1 illustrates the calculation for a 140 pound female with 30 percent body fat who wants to reduce to 20 percent body fat (80 percent fat-free weight). To determine goal weight, divide fat-free weight by 80 percent (.80), the fraction of the woman's goal weight that will be represented by fat-free weight. In this example the calculation provides a goal weight of 122.5 pounds . The woman must lose 17.5 pounds of body fat while maintaining her present amount of lean tissue to achieve 20 percent body fat.

Step #3: Determine Maintenance Caloric Needs

Energy requirements are determined by three components. *Resting (basal) metabolic rate (RMR)* represents the amount of energy required to support basic physiological functions such as breathing, pumping blood, and growing hair, to name a few. RMR accounts for 60 percent to 75 percent of the calories you burn each day. You will also use a certain amount of energy to digest the food that you eat. *The thermic effect of meals (TEM)* represents energy usage associated with digestion, absorption, transport and storage of digested food. TEM accounts for about 10 percent of your total energy expenditure each day. *Thermic effect of activity (TEA)* represents the energy expended for daily exercise, physical activity, and the like. Any estimation of average daily calorie needs will require you to make a few guesses pertaining to normal activity levels and lifestyle. As a consequence there will be a slight margin of error associated with any procedure.

✳ ***ACTION STEP: Determine Daily Calorie Needs.*** The following procedure can provide you with a fairly reliable estimate of your maintenance calorie needs. The calculation consists of four steps:

1. Estimate resting metabolic rate (RMR) by multiplying your body weight by 10.
2. Estimate the number of calories you burn, on average, for your workouts each day. For example, if you jog three mile per day add that number of calories to RMR.
3. Estimate the number of calories required to fuel daily activity apart from your workouts.
   - If you are sedentary estimate 20–40 percent RMR
   - If you are moderately active estimate 40–60 percent RMR
   - If you are very active estimate 60–80 percent RMR
4. Add steps 1, 2, and 3 to determine daily calorie requirement. *Adapted from Clark, 1997*

Step #4: Determine Rate of Fat Loss

Most experts agree that weight loss should be slow and steady. Table 12.2 illustrates the calorie deficit required to generate fat loss of one and two pounds per week, respectively.

TABLE 12.2: Caloric Deficit Required to Achieve Selected Rate of Fat Loss

To lose 1 pound per week, create deficit of 500 calories per day
To lose 2 pounds per week, create deficit of 1000 calories per day

Step #5: Create a Negative Energy Balance

A weight loss plan centered around regular exercise and a low-fat diet offers much greater flexibility that either method alone, and will enable you to remain in negative energy balance for extended periods of time. This is extremely important as studies demonstrate clearly that the greatest percentage of weight loss experienced during the first few days of a diet is due to water loss and depletion of carbohydrate stores. Substantially greater fat loss occurs only after you have stuck to the plan for several weeks. You can create a negative energy balance of 500 calories per day through moderate increases in physical activity coupled with smart food choices. A deficit of that magnitude will translate into a loss of one pound of fat per week.

* *ACTION STEP: Cut 250 calories daily.* You don't necessarily have to limit the amounts or types of food that you eat. Simply choose lower fat and/or lower calorie alternatives when possible. For example ...

Instead of these ...	Substitute these ...
French fries	Plain baked potato with pat of butter
Whole milk	1% milk
Ice Cream	Ice milk or sherbet
Caesar salad	Lettuce & tomato salad w/ vinegar & oil
Fried chicken	Skinless baked chicken
Steak	Broiled fish
Butter	Jelly or jam
Cream donut	English muffin
Soda Pop	Unsweetened ice tea
Whole eggs	Egg whites

* *ACTION STEP: Burn an additional 250 calories daily.* Performing one of the following every day will burn 250 additional calories ....

  - Walking for one hour
  - Jogging for 25 minutes
  - Cycling for 45 minutes
  - Gardening/digging for 30 minutes
  - Playing tennis for 40 minutes
  - Square dancing for 35 minutes
  - Skipping rope for 25 minutes

Note: You can burn an equivalent number of calories if you split the activity into two or three shorter segments. For example, take two 30-minute walks as opposed to one 60-minute walk.

Step #6: Rev Up Your Metabolism

Metabolism control can be an effective weight loss strategy, particularly when viewed over the long haul. Increase your resting metabolic rate and you will burn more calories, even during those times when you are just sitting around or sleeping. Over a period of time this can have a dramatic effect on body weight and body composition. Use the following strategies to jump start your metabolism.

* ***ACTION STEP: Weight train.*** You can condition your body to burn more calories by adding lean muscle. Strength training on two or three non-consecutive days per week can do this for you. Consider that an extra pound of muscle added to your frame will require an additional 30 to 50 calories per day to maintain. That can be the difference between gaining 3 or 4 pounds of fat in a year (30 or 40 pounds in a decade!) and maintaining normal weight.
* ***ACTION STEP: Regular aerobic exercise.*** Aerobic whole-body exercise will elevate your metabolic rate on a short-term basis. If the exercise is fairly vigorous your metabolism will remain elevated for a short time after the exercise

Lose Fat Through Functional Fitness

Practicing ***functional fitness*** can speed-up weight loss. Func tional fitness has a purpose above and beyond the exercise itself. For example, trimming the hedges and weeding the flower beds burns extra calories and also keeps your yard looking good. Substitute "body" work for "machine" work whenever possible. The following functional fitness activities burn about 100 calories.

- mowing the lawn for 25 minutes
- weeding the garden for 20 minutes
- washing windows for 30 minutes
- walking briskly for 20 minutes
- chopping wood for 15 minutes
- raking leaves for 25 minutes

has ended. Consider that burning an additional 100 calories per day (1 to 1 ½ mile walk) can translate into a fat loss of 10 pounds per year, assuming that eating and activity patterns remain constant.

✳ *ACTION STEP: Eat More Protein.* Increasing protein intake will elevate your metabolism slightly for the simple reason that digesting protein requires your body to expend more energy. I am not recommending that you adopt one of the popular high-protein high-fat diets currently on the market, nor do I suggest that you limit your intake of complex carbohydrates. You can combine carbohydrate-rich and low-fat protein-rich foods in the same meal.

✳ *ACTION STEP: Eat More Frequently.* Don't misinterpret this suggestion! I am not encouraging you to consume additional calories because that will surely lead to weight gain. Keep your daily caloric intake constant, but make an effort to consume those calories in smaller, more frequent meals spread throughout the day. Resting metabolic rate rises slightly after a meal, so eating more frequent meals will keep your metabolism elevated throughout the day. Eating four to six small meals per day will also keep you more satiated and make it less likely that you will gorge.

Step #7. Start Your Program TODAY!

The most important step of any journey is the one that gets you

Sample 8-Week Program to Lose Ten Pounds of Fat

(Create Caloric Deficit of 35,000 calories) 10 lb X 3500 cal/lb =35,000

	Calories		Total Cal
Weeks 1 & 2	Exercise = 250 calories/day X 8 days	2000	
	Diet = 400 calories/day X 14 days	5600	7600
Weeks 3 & 4	Exercise = 250 calories/day X 10 days	2500	
	Diet = 400 calories/day X 14 days	5600	8100
Weeks 5 & 6	Exercise = 300 calories/day X 10 days	3000	
	Diet = 400 calories/day X 14 days	5600	8600
Week 7 & 8	Exercise = 400 calories/day X 12 days	4800	
	Diet = 500 calories/day X 14 days	7000	11800
TOTAL	**36,100 cal**		

started. Take that step today. Identify your weight loss goals, create a plan you can live with and implement simple behavioral strategies that will gradually melt away the excess pounds. Small lifestyle changes consistently applied can result in significant physical change over the long haul. Inch by inch it's a cinch!

Getting Stronger 13

The first step in the process is to become familiar with the terminology. A *rep* is simply one repetition of an exercise. Re sistance training that creates maximal muscle tension with relatively few reps produces the greatest strength gains. Muscle endurance is developed using lighter resistance coupled with a greater number of reps. A ***set*** is a group of repetitions of an exercise; for example, one set of 10 reps. Healthy adult women beginning a program can start with one or possibly two sets of 8 to 12 reps per exercise.

Designing Your Program

A workout program customized to match your personal level of muscular fitness and long-term training goals is referred to as an *exercise prescription*. Research has identified specific prescriptions used to develop strength, endurance, tone and muscle definition. Improvements are stimulated by increasing the frequency of the movement (*repetitions*), the resistance to the movement *(weight)*, and/or the duration of the workout *(sets)*.

* **Exercise Selection.** During the early stages of your program focus on the development of total body strength rather than specific muscle groups. Strengthening the body core will provide a solid foundation for more specific muscle-shaping exercises later on. A complete workout should target the seven major muscle groups — chest, back, shoulders, biceps, triceps, legs and abs.

Add Muscle and Lose Inches?

In many cases getting stronger means getting smaller. Why? Be cause fat tissue is more bulky *(less dense)* than muscle. A pound of muscle takes up only about two-thirds as much space as a pound of fat. As muscle begins to replace fat, you may lose a size or two in clothing even though your body weight doesn't change significantly.

* **Exercise Order**. Target the largest muscle groups early in the workout. Perform exercises such as the bench press (chest), military press (shoulders), and pull downs (back) before curls (biceps) and push downs (triceps).
* **Exercise Frequency.** You should strength train every other day, or possibly every third day, to allow your muscles ample time between workouts for recovery. Competitive body builders seeking an edge may train more often. Strength workouts performed on consecutive days are usually centered around a "split routine" (different body parts exercised each day) or a "split program" (different exercises used for the same body part).
* **Exercise Volume**. Increase the total volume of exercise gradually and in small increments. You can do this by increasing the 1) number of sets performed, 2) number of repetitions per set, 3) and/or the resistance being moved.

NO PAIN, NO GAIN?

The "go for the burn" mentality is firmly entrenched in the fitness culture. Granted, exercise intensity is an important factor to consider when trying to improve muscular strength. You must overload the muscles for them to become stronger, so in that respect a feeling of discomfort should be considered a natural consequence of training. The feeling should be temporary, however, and quite different than a feeling of pain. Sharp pain is a warning signal that you are doing too much, too soon or too often.

Strength? Size? Tone?

There isn't a one-size-fits-all strength training program. To achieve maximum results you must identify your training goals and create a workout plan consistent with those aims. Consider the following guidelines when designing your workouts. Keep in mind that these are general recommendations only, and that there will always be a degree of overlap between programs.

To Develop Muscle Strength

1. Resistance: high (70-80% of your one-repetition maximum)
2. Repetitions per Set: 2 to 4

3. Sets: 3 to 5
4. Rest Between Sets: near full recovery (2 minutes or more)

To Develop Muscle Size

1. Resistance: moderate
2. Repetitions per Set: 4 to 8
3. Sets: 3 to 5
4. Rest Between Sets: partial recovery (30 to 90 seconds)

* *Note: Women will not experience the same degree of muscular hypertrophy as men.*

To Develop Muscle Tone

1. Resistance: light
2. Repetitions per Set: 12 to 20
3. Sets: 2 to 3
4. Rest Between Sets: very limited (30 to 60 seconds)

* *Note: If you are not comfortable developing a program on your own, I suggest you consult with a reputable certified personal trainer.*

What Type of Resistance Produces the Best Results?

Free Weights. Experienced lifters generally prefer to use free weights (dumbbells, barbells, bars and plates) to isolate and overload specific muscle groups. Free weight exercises provide a wide variety of lifting motions and, because the resistance is not attached to a machine, the lifter must maintain control of the weight throughout the entire range of motion. This balancing effect brings auxiliary muscle groups into play which adds to the total workout.

Resistance Machines. Machine-based exercise offers several advantages. Most machines are user-friendly and the movements require less skill than free-weight exercises. The lifter is guided through a specific range-of-motion with correct form, and the possibility of losing control of the weight has been eliminated. It is easy to adjust the resistance as you move from one machine to another, so workout time can be shortened. On the down side, machine-based exercises restrict you to a pre-designed set of lifts and movements, and you don' t learn to balance the load as well.

Manual Resistance. You can use your body weight as the resis-

Creatine

Muscle-Building Supplement or Myth?

Creatine occurs naturally in the body. It is produced in the liver and the kidneys from non-essential amino acids. Some creatine is stored in muscle cells where it is turned into a compound called creatine phosphate (CP) which functions as a miniature energy supply for the muscles. CP is particularly important for activities that require short, explosive bursts of activity, such as weight training. CP also functions to restock cellular reserves of ATP, the energy fuel that provides the impetus for muscular contraction. Unlike many of the muscle-building supplements on the market, the effects of creatine supplementation on strength development has been researched fairly extensively. Findings suggest that creatine taken in conjunction with strength training can produce significant improvement in levels of strength and power.

Creatine does not build muscle directly. When you load additional creatine into your muscles it enables you to train longer and harder. Your muscles will also recover more quickly from the workouts. The fact that you can workout more frequently and with greater intensity is what actually results in the additional muscle and strength gains. You still have to do the work! Although some people have complained of muscle cramping in conjunction with creatine usage, others have not reported any short-term negative effects. The long-term effects of creative supplementation are unknown.

tance to be moved. Push-ups, pull-ups, dips, step-ups, lunges, crunches and isometric exercises offer the advantage of convenience, no cost, and a high degree of safety. There are minor drawbacks. You are limited insofar as the types of exercises, and it is not possible to adjust the resistance to any great extent. To work your muscles to the point of momentary fatigue will require you to manipulate the number of reps and/or number of sets.

The Verdict? When all is said and done your muscles really don't know the difference between the resistance supplied by a dumbbell, a machine, your own body weight, or a bucket of sand for that matter. A much more important consideration is the consistency and intensity of your workouts. Towards that aim you should select exercises that are relatively convenient to do and movements that you are willing to perform on a regular basis.

More Protein ... More Muscles?

The benefits of protein supplementation have been greatly ex aggerated. While protein does play an important role in the growth and repair of cells, excessive protein intake is of no real benefit and can actually be hazardous to your health. Supplementing your diet with huge amounts of protein will not add muscle to your frame. Only strength training can do that.

Training Guidelines

The American College of Sports Medicine recommends the following weight-training guidelines for normal healthy adult women.

- ✳ Select 8 to 10 exercises that target the major muscle groups.
- ✳ Streamline your program. Workouts lasting longer than 1 hour are associated with higher dropout rates.
- ✳ Perform one or more sets of 8 to12 repetitions for each exercise to the point of momentary fatigue
- ✳ Perform workouts at least 2 times per week on non-consecutive days
- ✳ Perform each exercise through a full range-of-motion
- ✳ Perform both the lifting **(concentric phase)** and lowering **(eccentric phase)** portion of the exercises in a controlled manner
- ✳ Maintain a normal breathing pattern. Holding your breath can cause a significant increase in blood pressure
- ✳ Exercise with a training partner who can provide assistance and motivation

Tips for Beginners

One of every two beginning exercisers dropout during the first month or two of a new program. If you are just getting started the following tips will help to keep you motivated during those critical first few weeks ...

- ✳ **Light is Right.** Choose a weight you can lift 12 to15 repetitions, but perform only 8 to 10 repetitions. Gradually increase the resistance to make your workouts more challenging.

* **One Set is Best.** One set per exercise may be sufficient during the beginning stages of a program. It doesn't make much sense to jump from zero sets (prior to beginning your program) to three sets per exercise. Your goal is to overload the muscle, not bury it!
* **Differentiate Between Pain and Soreness.** You should expect to experience some soreness during the initial stages of a weight-training program. Extreme discomfort is a different story. Stop exercising immediately if you feel sharp pain during or after a workout.
* **Take It Inch by Inch.** Progressive overloading of the muscles is the key to continued improvement. As muscles get stronger adjust the resistance as needed to maintain a weight that you can lift 8 to 12 repetitions. Eventually increase the number of sets per exercise as well.

The Home Gym

Lack of time is an oft-cited reason for failure to stick with an exercise program. One possible solution is a home gym. Your personal in-home health club can provide the ultimate in exercise convenience. You've eliminated the travel time to and from the club. You can listen to music or catch up on the evening news as you workout on the stationary bike. You can exercise early or late, whenever it fits into your daily schedule. The "club" is open 24 hours a day.

Safe Lifting

Resistance training is a very safe activity when performed correctly. You can minimize the likelihood of injury by adhering to the following safety guidelines.

* **Breathing.** Blood pressure can rise substantially when lifting weights, which makes the heart work harder. Holding your breath will compound the problem by closing the glottis which functions as a safety valve that can relieve pressure. To avoid this problem you should exhale during the lifting phase of the exercise and inhale during the lowering phase.

- ✳ **Spotting**. A training partner (spotter) is recommended when training with heavy free weights. The spotter can assist in controlling the weight and also help you to safely perform extra repetitions of an exercise. A competent spotter should possess sufficient strength to assist you if needed, be familiar with the proper spotting technique, pay attention at all times, and be aware of how many repetitions you are going to attempt.
- ✳ **Proper Lifting Technique**. Correct form will maximize strength gains and prevent unnecessary injury. Most weight training injuries are due to the lifter attempting to move a resistance that exceeds her or his strength capabilities.

Plyometric Training

Plyometric exercises combine elements of strength and speed training to develop increased power and explosiveness. Movements required for sports such as basketball, soccer, and track involve sudden changes in muscle length. For example, changing speed and direction while dribbling a basketball involves lengthening *(eccentric)* muscle contractions followed rapidly by shortening *(concentric)* contractions. The more quickly the concentric contraction follows the eccentric contraction, the greater the power generated. Plyometric training is designed to speed up the *eccentric-concentric contraction* which in turn enhances your ability for explosive-type movement. Plyometric exercises involve rapid changes of direction such as hopping, bounding, jumping or skipping. Because such movements place a great deal of stress on muscles and connective tissues they are not appropriate for most people.

Shaping a Feminine Physique 14

There isn't a generic cookbook-type strength training program guaranteed to produce results for everyone. You must take into account your present physical condition, identify and prioritize your training goals, and then put together a workout designed to achieve those aims. It is my experience that most women are more interested in toning, tightening and reshaping their body than they are in simply becoming as strong as possible. If that general observation applies to your situation consider the following:

Train with high reps. A range between 12 to 20 reps per exercise is about right for most women. Training with high reps targets your slow-twitch (endurance) muscle fibers which have limited ability to grow larger, so you won't end up with big bulky muscles. Your muscles will develop tone however, and become more shapely and defined. Training with higher reps also burns more calories than training with low reps, which will help to decrease body fat stores.

Keep rest intervals short. To create maximal stress on the targeted muscles keep the rest intervals between sets at a minimum, generally between 30 and 60 seconds. By not allowing your muscles to fully recover between sets you add an aerobic component to your strength program. This keeps your heart rate slightly elevated and allows for increased energy expenditure.

Train hard. There are no shortcuts to sculpting a shapely feminine physique. You must push your muscles beyond the point of effort that they are normally accustomed to, and you must do this on a regular basis. For best results you should take each set to the point of momentary fatigue, the point where you can't do another rep. For this reason a training partner should be present to assist in all exercises.

Kim King, strength and conditioning specialist at the University of Pittsburgh, has provided the following strength-training programs based on the lifter's level of expertise and experience. These prescriptions are provided as examples only and should be adapted to accommodate your specific training goals

Basic Beginner Lifting Program

This is a three-day workout program, and it is suggested that it be done every other day. This same workout can be advanced after 2–4 weeks simply by increasing your number of sets to 3 and your repetitions to 12–15.

Day One

Movements	Set x Reps
Warm-up	
Chest press machine or incline dumbbell press	2 x 10
Peck deck machine or incline dumbbell fly	2 x 10
Lat pull to front using a shoulder width grip	2 x 10
One arm DB row	2 x 10
Seated low cable row	2 x 10
Back extension	2 x 10
Abdominals: Bent knee sit-up	2 x 10
Hip-up	2 x 10

Day Two

Movements	Set x Reps
Warm-up	
Back squat	2 x 10
Leg press	2 x 10
Leg extension	2 x 10
Dumbbell lunges	2 x 10
Lying or seated leg curl	2 x 10
Seated calf raise	2 x 10
Abdominals: Crunches	2 x 10
Lying bent knee leg raise	2 x 10

Day Three

Movements	Set x Reps
Warm-up	
Shoulder press machine or seated DB shoulder press	2 x 10
Side DB lateral raise	2 x 10
Seated bent over DB rear lateral raise	2 x 10
Standing tricep push down	2 x 10
Standing bicep machine curls	2 x 10
Standing DB bicep curls	2 x 10
Abdominals: Crunches	2 x 10
Incline leg pull-in	2 x 10

Basic Intermediate Lifting Program

This is a three-day workout program, and it is suggested that it be done every other day. This would be considered a toning program

Day One

Movements	Set x Reps
Warm-up	
Back squats	3 x 15
Leg extensions	3 x 20
Lying or seated leg curl	3 x 15
Dumbbell lunges	3 x 15
Seated dumbbell shoulder press	3 x 15
Side dumbbell lateral raise	3 x 15
Abdominals: Bent knee sit-up	3 x 30
Hip-up	3 x 30

Day Two

Movements	Set x Reps
Warm-up	
Chest press machine	3 x 12
Incline dumbbell press	3 x 15
Incline dumbbell fly	3 x 15
Lat pull-down to front	3 x 15
Seated low cable row	3 x 15
Back extensions	3 x 15
Abdominals: Crunches	3 x 30
Lying bent knee leg raise	3 x 20

Day Three

Movements	Set x Reps
Warm-up	
Leg press	3 x 15
Dumbbell step up	3 x 12
Walking dumbbell lunges	3 x 12 steps
Lying or seated leg curl	3 x 15
Tricep cable push-down	3 x 15
Bicep cable curls	3 x 15
Bench dips	3 x failure
Abdominals: Toe touch crunches	3 x 30
Incline leg pull-in	3 x 20

Advanced Lifting Program

This workout is called a superset style (SS) workout; it develops tone and shape. Supersets are done by performing two movements directly after another without rest.

Day One

Movements		Set x Reps
Warm up		
Squat SS/with DB straight leg dead lift		3 x 15/15
Alternating DB step up SS/with alternating DB lunges		3 x 16/16
Lying leg curl SS/with seated leg curl		3 x 15/15
Incline DB chest press SS/ with incline DB fly		3 x 15/15
Abdominals:	Bent knee sit-up	3 x 30
	Lying toe touch	3 x 30
	Right crunch	3 x 30
	Left crunch	3 x 30
	Hip-up	3 x 30

Day Two

Movements		Set x Reps
Warm up		
Seated DB shoulder press SS/with upright cable row		3 x 15/15
Front/side DB shoulder lateral raise		3 x 12/12
Bent over DB lateral raise SS/with strap pulls to chin		3 x 15/15
Tricep push down SS/with bench dips		3 x 15/15
Bicep cable curls SS/with DB bicep curls		3 x 15/15
Abdominals:	Bent knee sit-up	3 x 30
	Lying bent knee leg raise	3 x 30

Day Three

Movements		Set x Reps
Warm-up		
Leg press SS/with leg extensions		3 x 15/15
Walking DB lunges SS/with leg extensions		3 x 16 steps/15
Seated leg curl SS/with back extensions		3 x 15/15
Lat pull to fron SS/with low cable row		3 x 15/15
Abdominals:	Circuit style	3 x 30
	Toe touch crunch	3 x 30
	Crunch twist	3 x 30
	Hip-up	3 x 30

Lifting Program for Size and Strength

This workout is for an advanced lifter and should be done with a spotter. It is a three day per week workout.

Day One

Movements	**Set x Reps**
Warm-up	
Flat bench press	3 x 4/3/2
Incline dumbbell press	3 x 6
Incline dumbbell fly	3 x 6
One arm dumbbell row	3 x 6/4/4
Lat pull to front–vary grips	3 x 8
Low cable rows	3 x 6

Day Two

Movements	**Set x Reps**
Warm-up	
Seated front military press	4 x 6/4/3/2
Side dumbbell lateral raise	3 x 6
Standing bent over dumbbell lateral raise	3 x 6
Lying tricep extension	3 x 6/4/4
Tricep push down	3 x 6
Standing bicep straight bar curls	3 x 6

Day Three

Movements	**Set x Reps**
Warm-up	
Back squat	4 x 6/4/3/2
Leg press	3 x 8/6/6
Leg extension	3 x 10
Lying or seated leg curl	3 x 8
Standing calf raise	3 x 8

Strength Training Exercises

A variety of exercises can be used to tone, tighten and reshape your body. The following examples are provided to assist in designing your personal program. Exercises are grouped according to the major muscle groups involved in the lift.

CHEST

Straight Bar Flat Bench Press (Free Weight)

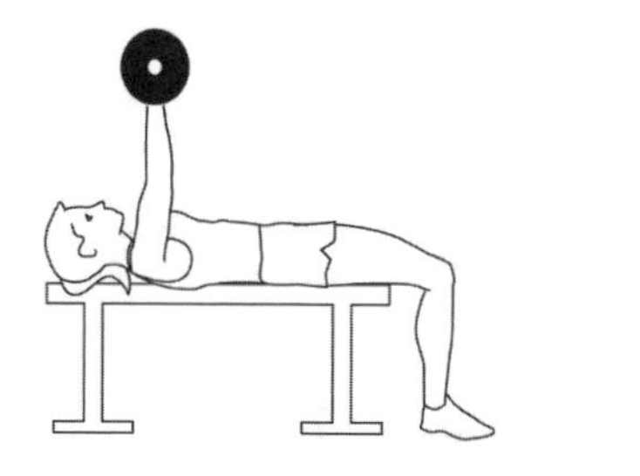

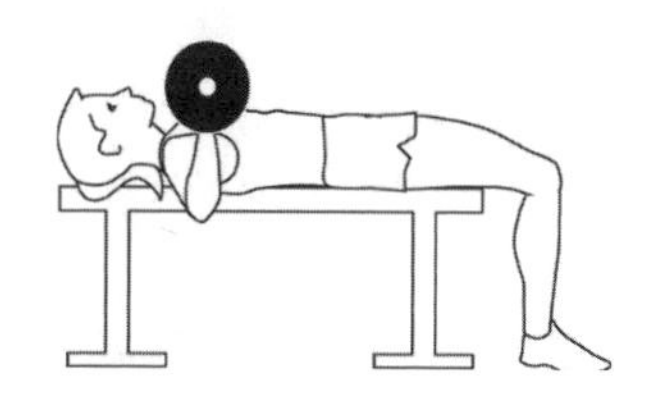

- Lie flat on your back with shoulders and buttocks in contact with the bench.
- Plant feet firmly on ground.
- Grasp bar with an overhand grip with hands about 6 inches wider than shoulders.
- Lift bar off of bar shelf (assisted by spotter) and position it over your chest with arms fully extended.
- Slowly lower bar to chest; do not bounce bar off of chest.
- Push weight back up to full elbow extension; do not arch back and do not raise buttocks off of bench.
- Inhale on the downward movement; exhale while raising the bar.

Dumbbell Flat Bench Press (Free Weight)

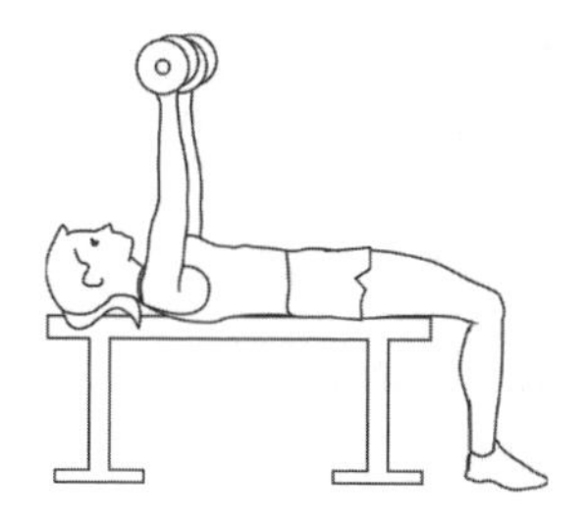

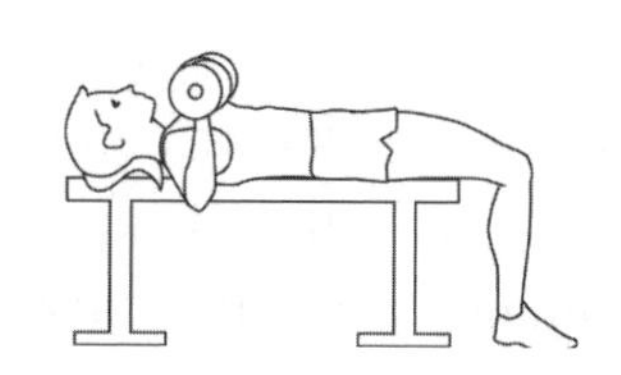

- Lie flat on bench with your feet on floor.
- Hold dumbbells at arms length directly above shoulders with palms facing forward.
- Slowly lower the dumbbells until they are even with and 12 inches to each side of your chest.
- Return dumbbells to starting position using same path.
- Inhale while lowering; exhale while raising.

Chest Press Machine

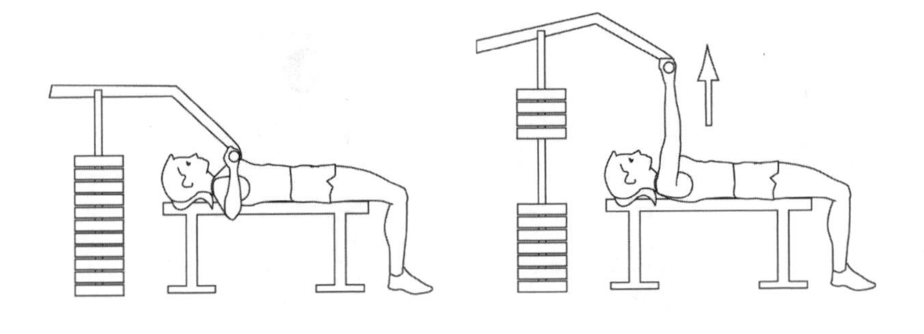

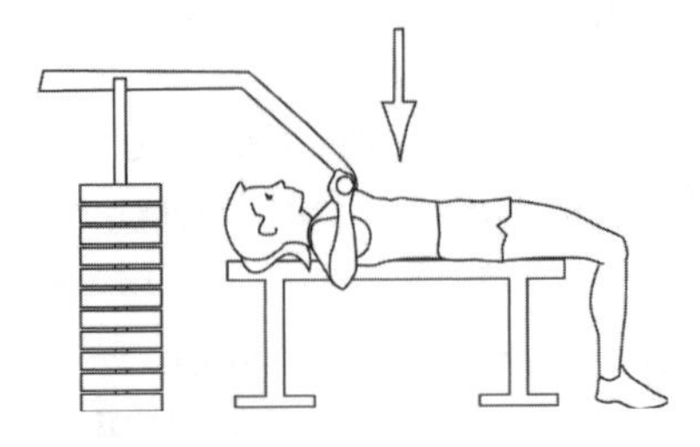

- Lie face up on the bench with feet straddling the bench and flat on the floor.
- Grasp handles slightly wider than shoulders with a closed overhand grip.
- Align handles with center chest.
- Push handles upward to a fully extended elbow position.
- Keep feet flat on floor and do not arch lower back.
- Lower the weight slowly and under control.
- Exhale during the upward lifting motion.
- Inhale during the downward phase.

Straight Bar Incline Bench Press (Free Weight)

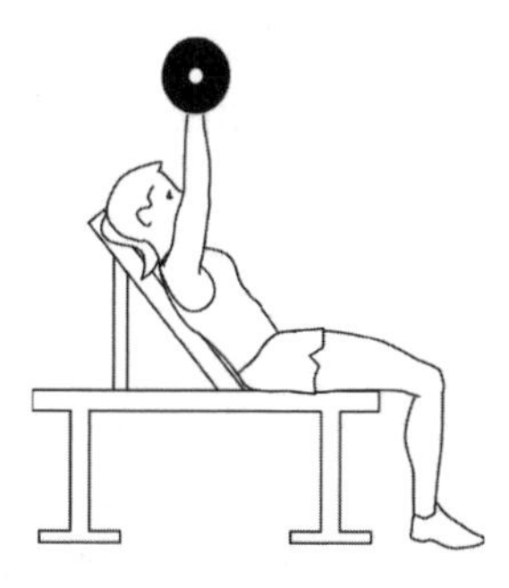

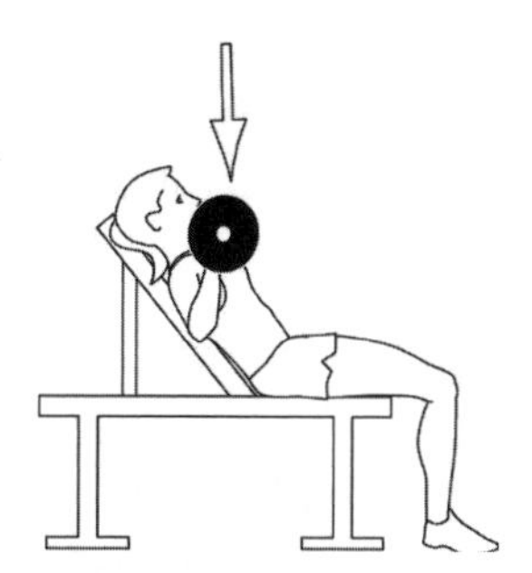

- ✳ Lie facing forward on the incline bench.
- ✳ Grasp bar with hands slightly wider than shoulder width apart.
- ✳ Keep back flat against incline bench with feet firmly planted on floor.
- ✳ Lift bar off of shelf *(assisted by spotter)* and position weight directly above upper chest.
- ✳ Slowly lower weight to upper chest.
- ✳ Pause, focus eyes upward, drive through legs, and push weight up to starting position.
- ✳ Keep head on bench throughout motion; do not arch back too sharply.
- ✳ Do not raise hips off of bench.
- ✳ Inhale during downward movement; exhale during upward movement.

Flat Bench Dumbbell Fly (Free Weight)

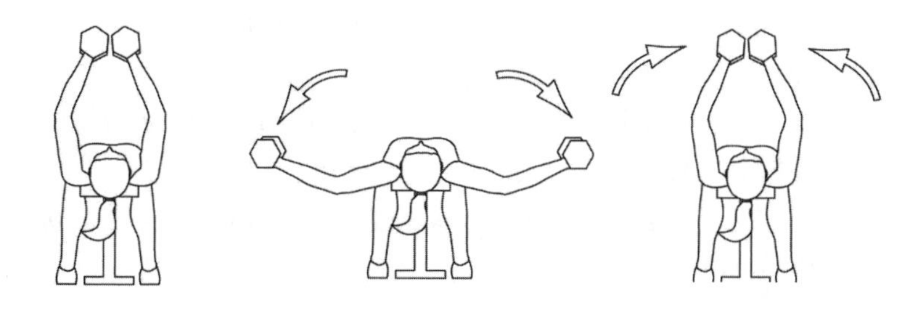

- Lie face up on bench with feet on floor.
- Grasp dumbbells and position them above chest with arms extended.
- Rotate dumbbells so that palms face one other.
- Point elbows out.
- Flex elbows slightly.
- Move dumbbells outward in wide arc.
- Keep dumbbells in line with shoulders while lowering them to shoulder level.
- To raise, pull dumbbells evenly toward each other in a wide arc until they reach a position above your chest.
- Keep elbows slightly flexed until reaching starting position.
- Inhale during downward movement; exhale during upward movement phase.

Push-ups (Manual resistance)

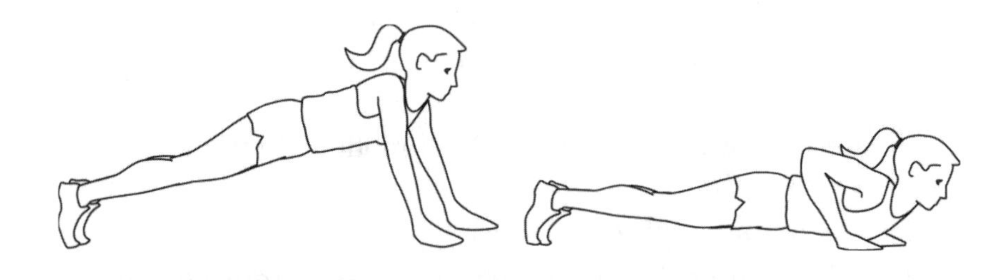

- Assume push-up position with arms approximately shoulder-width apart.
- Keep back straight and legs fully extended behind you.
- Slowly lower your body until chest touches the ground.
- Do not let your body sag.
- Push upward with arms and return to starting position.
- Inhale while lowering; exhale while rising.

  NOTE: Beginners can do modified push-ups (weight supported on knees).

SHOULDERS

Straight Bar Shoulder Press (Free Weights)

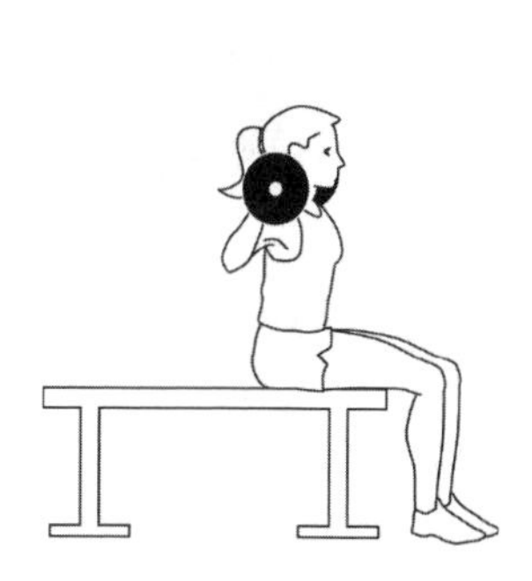

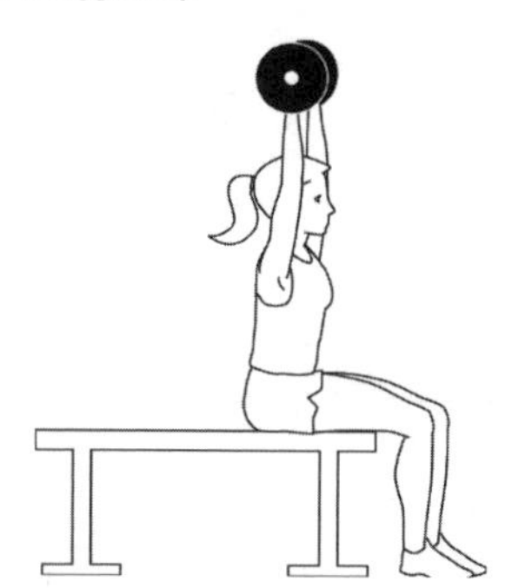

- ✳ Sit on military bench with back straight.
- ✳ Grasp bar with overhand grip slightly wider than shoulder width.
- ✳ Lift bar off of rack (assisted by spotter) and slowly lower to chest.
- ✳ Begin upward movement with bar positioned on upper chest.
- ✳ Drive through legs and lift bar straight up.
- ✳ Press bar to arms length overhead.
- ✳ Pause for a moment, then slowly lower bar to upper chest.
- ✳ Rest bar on chest between reps.
- ✳ Inhale during the downward movement, exhale through sticking point of upward movement.

  NOTE: *You can perform this exercise using dumbbells instead of a straight bar. The shoulder press exercise can also be performed in the standing position*

Shoulder Press (Machine)

- ✳ Sit on stool and grasp handles with overhand grip.
- ✳ Keep back straight and position feet on floor (on or rungs of the stool).
- ✳ Focus eyes straight ahead.

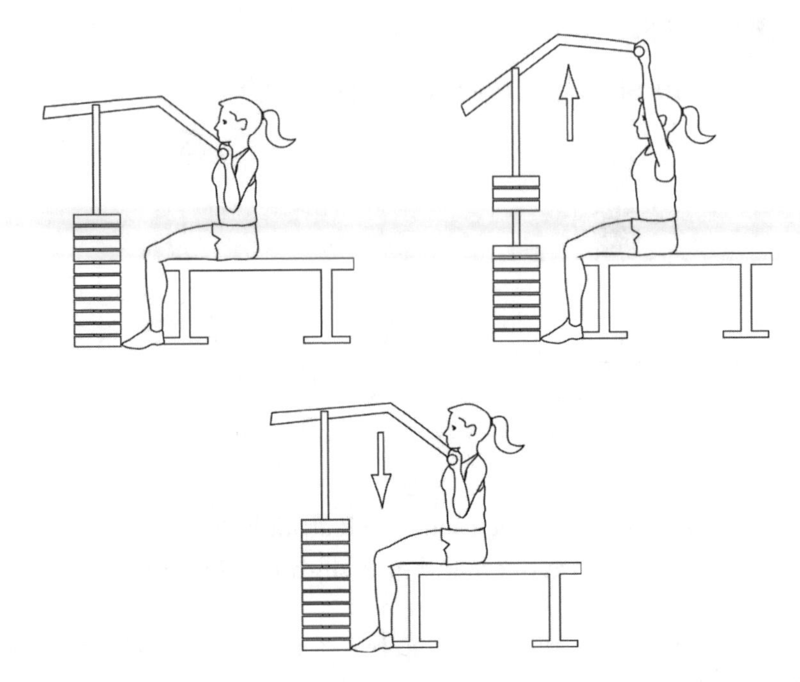

* Push handles up, keep elbows pointed out to sides until arms are fully extended.
* Pause, then lower handles slowly and under control to shoulder level.
* Do not jerk or bounce.
* Inhale during downward movement, exhale through sticking point of upward movement.

Lateral Side Raise (Free Weights)

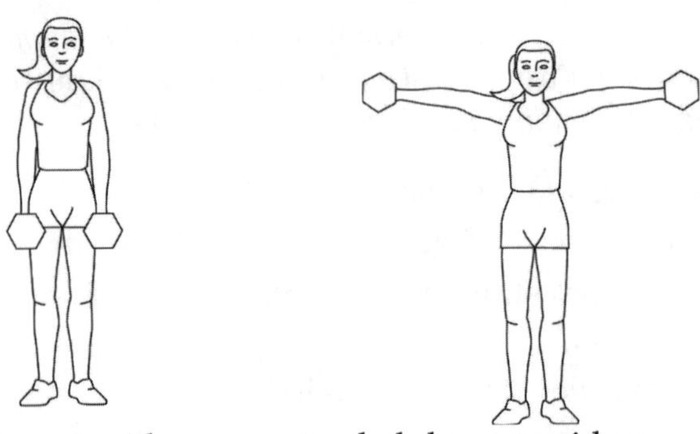

* Stand erect with arms extended down to sides.

- ✳ Hold dumbbells with palms facing in.
- ✳ Raise dumbbells in a semicircular motion to a position slightly above shoulder height.
- ✳ Pause, lower dumbbells to starting position using same pathway.
- ✳ Keep arms straight as you raise dumbbells.
- ✳ Inhale while lowering; exhale while raising weight.

Note: This exercise can also be done when seated on lateral raise machine.

Shoulder Shrug (Free Weights)

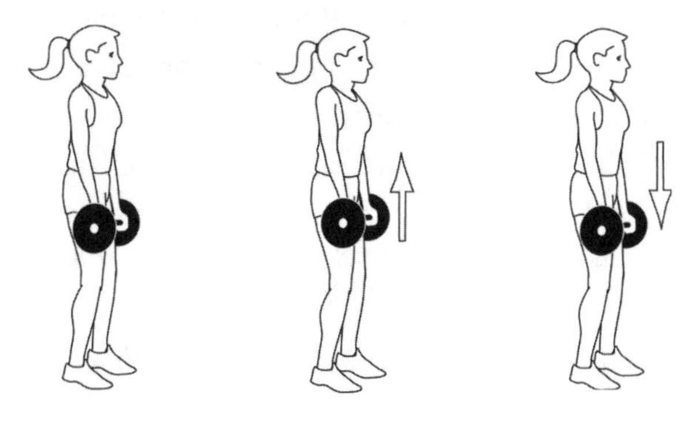

- ✳ Grasp bar in pronated grip with hands shoulder-width apart.
- ✳ Assume upright starting position.
- ✳ Feet shoulder-width apart with knees flexed slightly.
- ✳ Arms fully extended down.
- ✳ Raise bar by elevating shoulders toward ears.
- ✳ Keep elbows fully extended and maintain upright posture.
- ✳ Shrug shoulders as high as possible.
- ✳ Lower bar slowly, pause, and repeat.
- ✳ Inhale during downward movement; exhale during sticking point of upward movement.

Dumbbell Front Raise (Free weights)

- ✳ Stand holding dumbbells in front of your thighs with palms facing in.

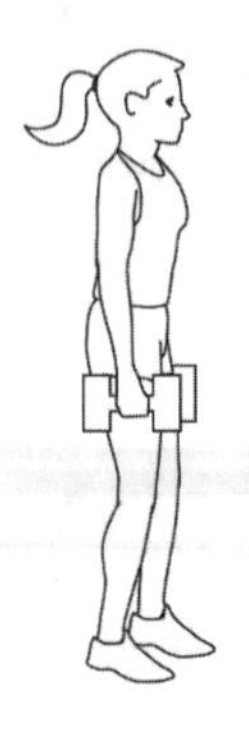
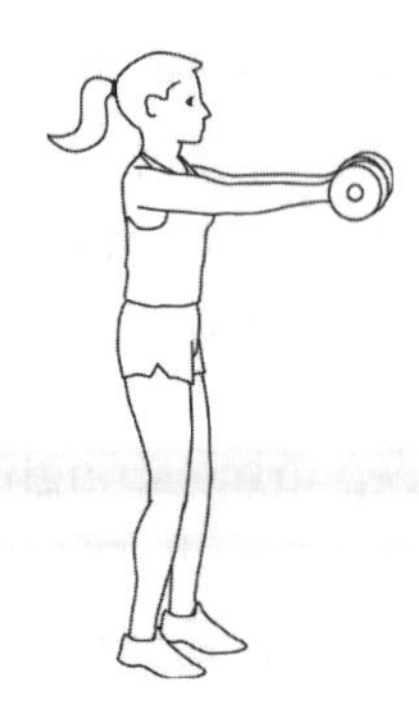

* Position feet shoulder-width apart with knees slightly flexed.
* Keep arms extended with elbows slightly bent.
* Raise dumbbells in an arc until arms are parallel to floor.
* Return dumbbells to starting position using same pathway.
* Exhale during downward movement; inhale during upward movement.

  Note: This exercise can be performed when sitting and by alternating one arm up, one arm down.

Bentover Dumbbell Lateral Raise (Free Weights)

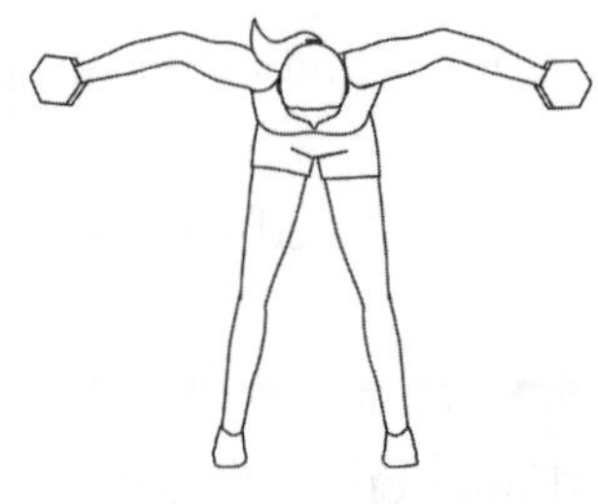
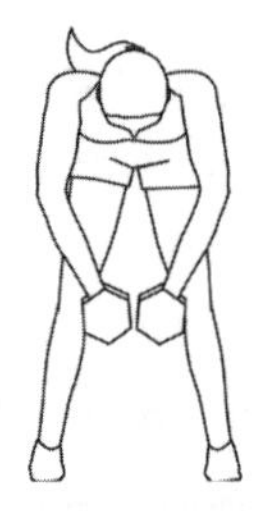

* Flex your knees slightly and lean forward from the waist.
* Your upper torso should be parallel with the floor.
* Keep your back perfectly flat; not rounded.
* Your arms hang straight down holding dumbbells.
* With elbows slightly flexed raise the dumbbells laterally and upward until your arms are slightly higher than parallel with the floor.
* Exhale when raising your arms.

- Slowly lower your arms until they are perpendicular to the floor.
- Inhale when lowering your arms.

BACK

Medium Grip Pull-ups (Manual Resistance)

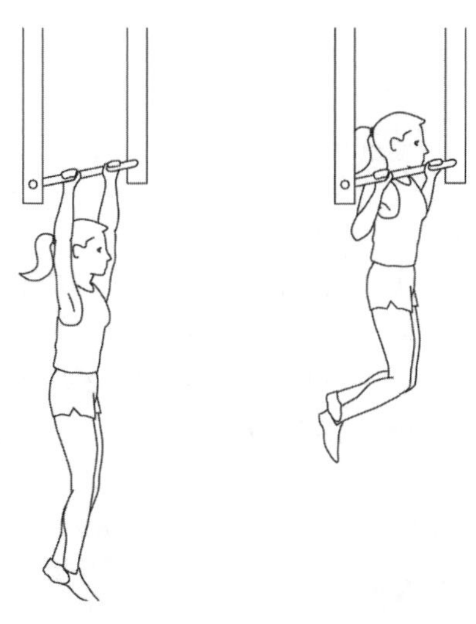

- Grip bar with overhand grip and hands approximately shoulder-width apart.
- Hang on chin up bar with legs fully extended beneath you.
- Pull body upward in controlled movement until chin is even with bar.
- Slowly lower body to starting position.
- Do not swing back and forth.
- Exhale while lowering body; inhale while raising body.
- Repeat as many times as possible.

  Note: Variations use close hand grip, wide grip, reverse grip (palms facing inward).

Front Lat Pull-Down (Machine)

- Kneel down facing machine.
- Grasp bar in overhand grip with hands wider than shoulder-width.

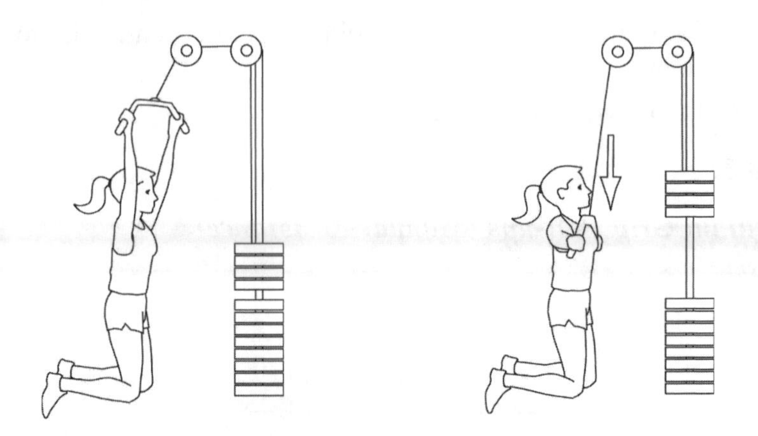

- Arms should be fully extended.
- Pull bar straight down in front of your face until it touches the base of your neck just above the chest.
- Pause, then slowly return to starting position.
- Inhale will pulling weight downward; exhale while raising weight.

Note: This exercise can also be done with medium-width grip.

One Arm Dumbbell Row (Free Weights)

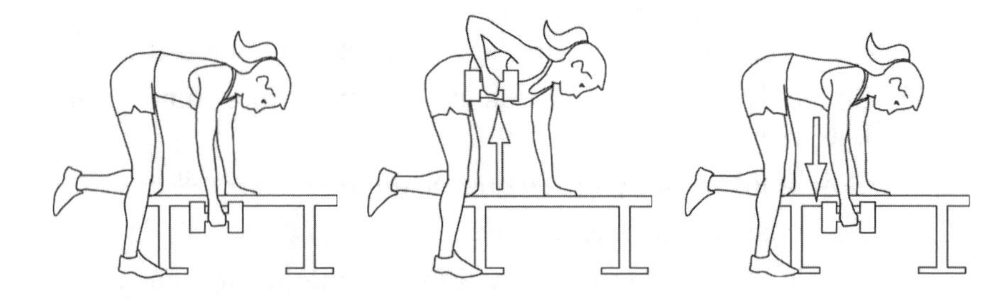

- Stand on one side of a weight bench.
- Kneel on bench with your inside leg.
- Plant outside leg beside bench with knee flexed.
- Lean forward and place inside hand on the bench in front of your inside leg.
- Position back parallel to floor and grasp dumbbell with outside hand.

* Elbow should be fully extended.
* Pull dumbbell upward to touch outer chest and rib cage.
* Lower dumbbell slowly and under control until elbow fully extended.
* Keep upper arm and elbow close to ribs.
* Exhale when lifting weight; inhale during downward movement.

Seated Cable Row (Machine)

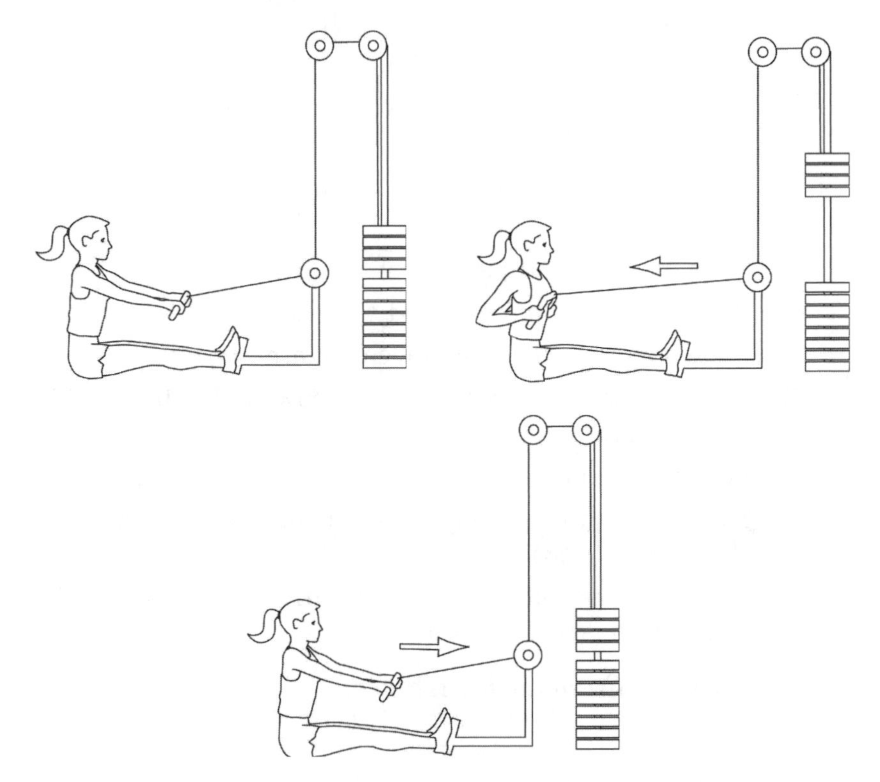

* Sit facing machine with knees flexed and feet against support platform.
* Lean forward and grab cable handles with arms fully extended.
* Pull the cable handle to the sides of your chest in line with pectorals.
* Do not rock or lean backwards.

- Pause, slowly return arms to fully extended starting position.
- Keep elbows next to ribs throughout motion.
- Exhale when pulling weight towards you; inhale when returning weight to start position.

Pullover (Machine)

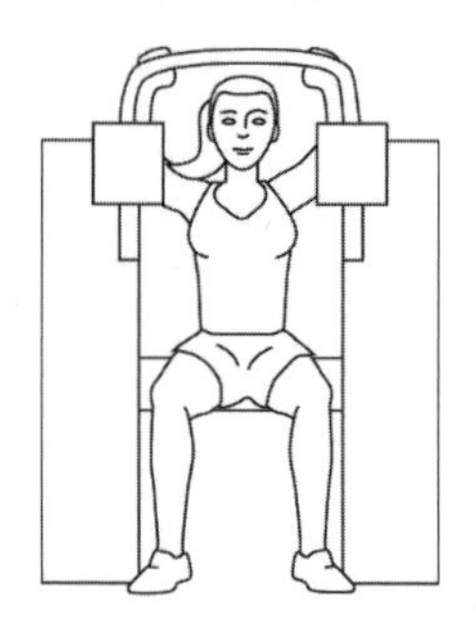

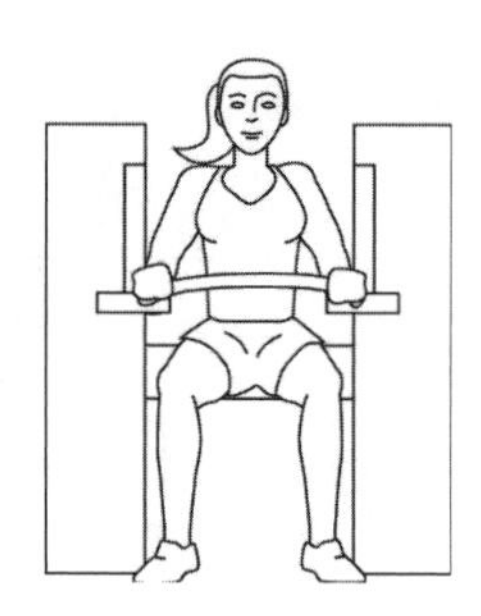

- Sit in machine and fasten seat belt.
- Place elbows on pads behind your head.
- Place hands against the movement arm.
- Pull down bar by pushing with elbows rather than pulling with hands.
- Pull movement arm to mid-section during every repetition.
- Slowly return to starting position (elbows near or slightly above your head).
- Exhale when pulling movement arm down; inhale when returning to starting position.

Back Extension (Manual Resistance)

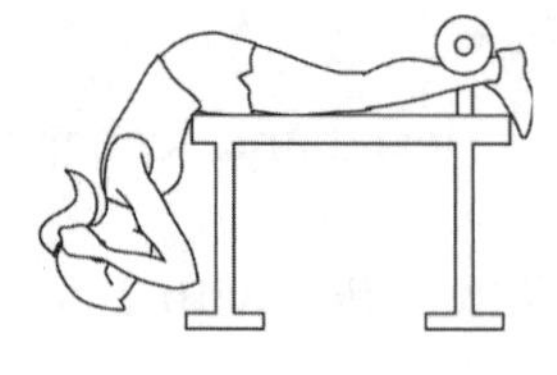

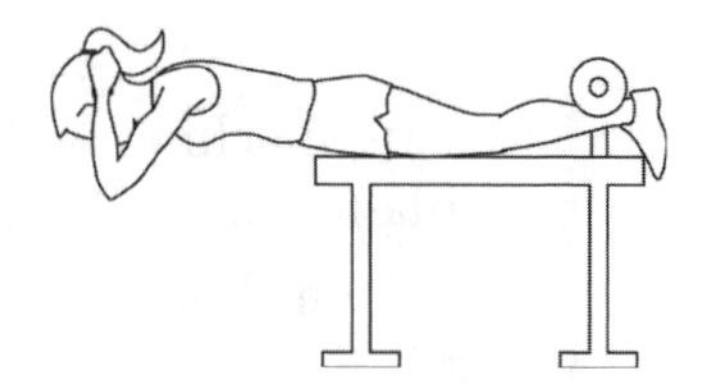

- Assume a prone position supported at the waist.
- Allow your upper body to extend off of the bench.

- ✳ Make sure your heels are held securely in place by the machine (or a training partner).
- ✳ Place your hands behind your neck or across your chest.
- ✳ Slowly lower your upper body to a position perpendicular to the floor.
- ✳ Inhale as you lower your body.
- ✳ Raise your upper torso back to the starting position and hold that position momentarily before repeating the exercise.
- ✳ Exhale as you return to the starting position.

ARMS

Straight Bar Bicep Curl (Free Weights)

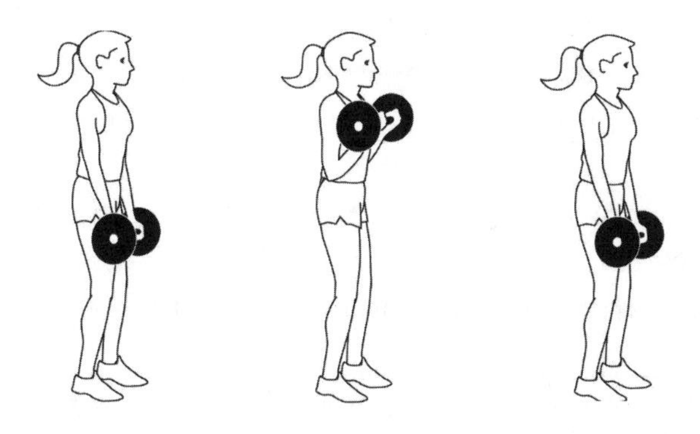

- ✳ Hold bar with hands approximately 12 inches apart and palms facing up.
- ✳ Stand erect with back straight and feet shoulder-width apart.
- ✳ Begin with bar at arms length resting against upper thighs.
- ✳ Position upper arms against ribs and perpendicular to the floor.
- ✳ Curl the bar upward in a semi-circular motion by flexing arms at the elbow until forearms touch bicep.
- ✳ Keep upper arms and elbows stationary; do not swing the weight up.
- ✳ Lower your arms slowly until elbows fully extended.

* Exhale during sticking point of the upward movement; inhale during downward movement.

Hammer Bicep Curl (Free Weights)

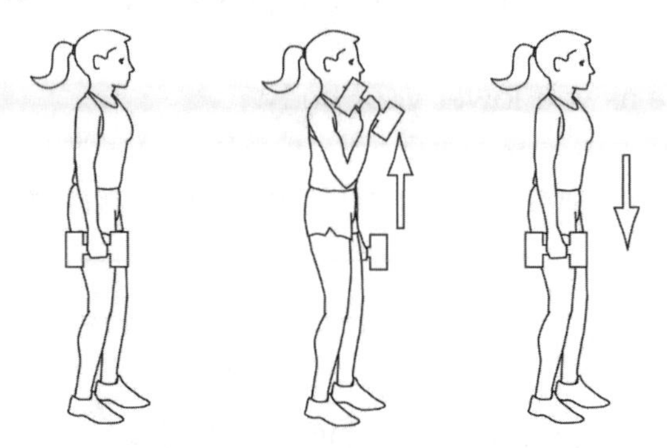

* Stand erect with feet shoulder width apart.
* Hold dumbbells with arms extended downward to sides.
* Palms should be facing inward toward outer thighs.
* Position upper arms against ribs and perpendicular to the floor.
* Raise one dumbbell at a time by flexing the arm at the elbow.
* Upward movement should bring dumbbell in line with shoulder.
* Lower dumbbell slowly until elbow is fully extended.
* Repeat upward and downward movement with opposite arm.
* Exhale during upward movement phase; inhale during downward phase.

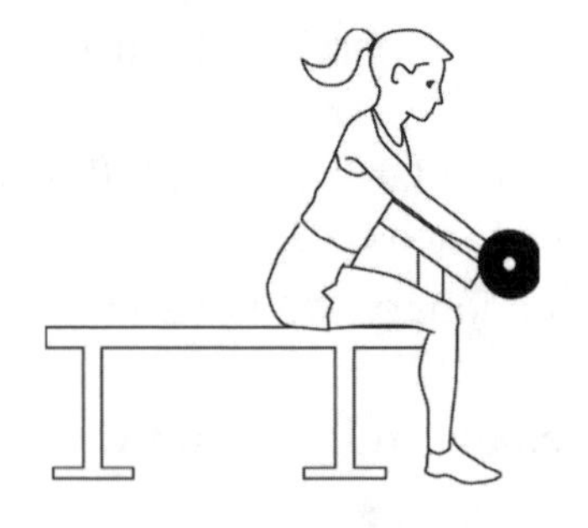

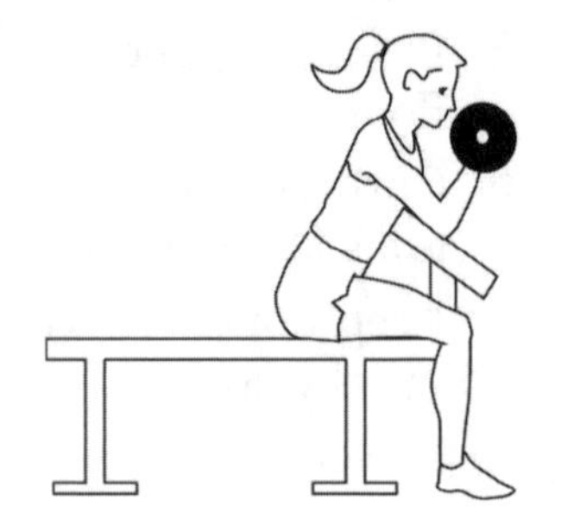

Preacher Bicep Curl (Free Weights)

- ✳ Sit facing forward on a preacher bench with chest and arms against pad.
- ✳ Extend upper pectorals over the end of the bench.
- ✳ Grip bar with palms facing upward and hands approximately 15 inches apart.
- ✳ Keep upper arms (triceps) against pad.
- ✳ Start with elbows extended and bar at arms length
- ✳ Curl bar in semicircular motion until forearms touch biceps.
- ✳ Slowly return bar to starting position using same path.
- ✳ Do not allow elbows to go beyond full extension position.
- ✳ Exhale during upward movement, inhale while lowering bar.

Triceps Push-down (Machine)

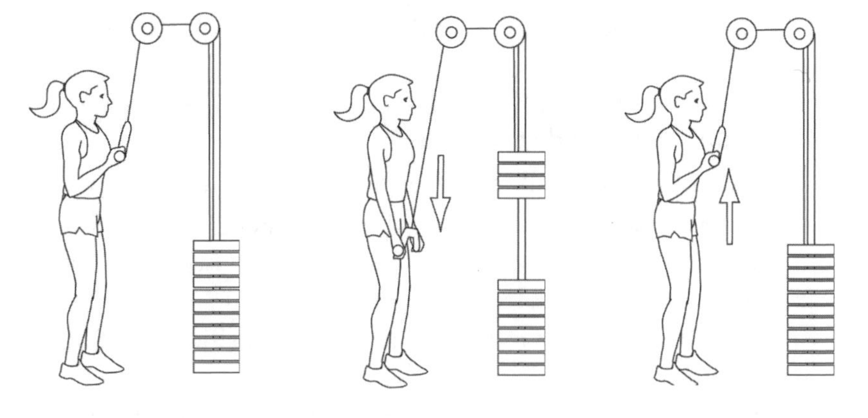

- ✳ Stand erect facing bar with feet shoulder-width apart.
- ✳ Grasp bar in an overhand grip with hands close together.
- ✳ Begin with elbows tight to sides and bar at mid-chest height.
- ✳ Push bar downward to full elbow extension.
- ✳ Avoid leaning forward into bar.
- ✳ Allow bar to rise to starting position, slowly and under control.
- ✳ Elbows should remain motionless throughout the movement.

Lying Triceps Extension (Free Weights)

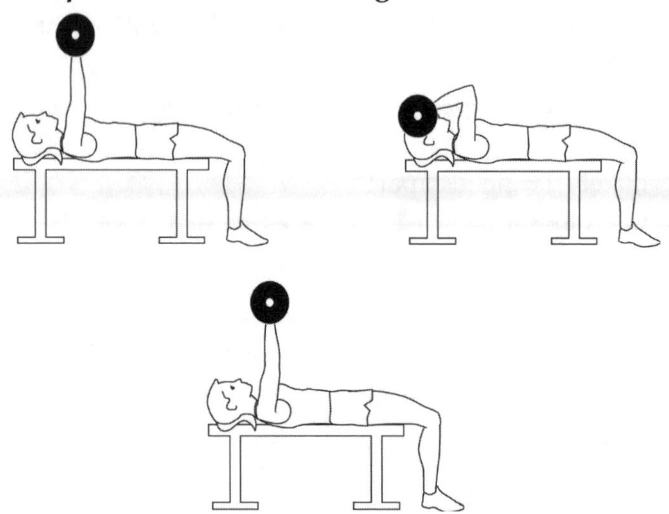

- ✳ Lie flat on your back on the bench.
- ✳ Rest your head on one end of the bench with feet flat on floor.
- ✳ Grasp the bar with palms facing up and hands approximately thumbs distance apart.
- ✳ Extend arms to full length directly above chest.
- ✳ Keep upper arms perpendicular to the bench as you flex at the elbows and lower the bar to a position just above your forehead.
- ✳ Pause, then slowly return bar to starting position using same path.
- ✳ Inhale during downward movement phase; exhale through sticking point of upward movement phase.

Bench Dips (Manual Resistance)

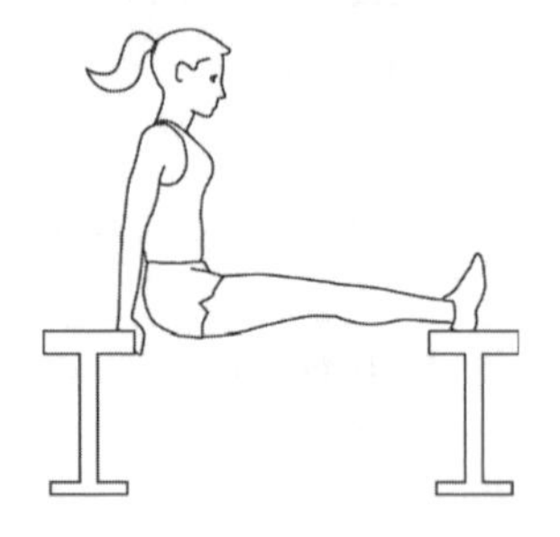

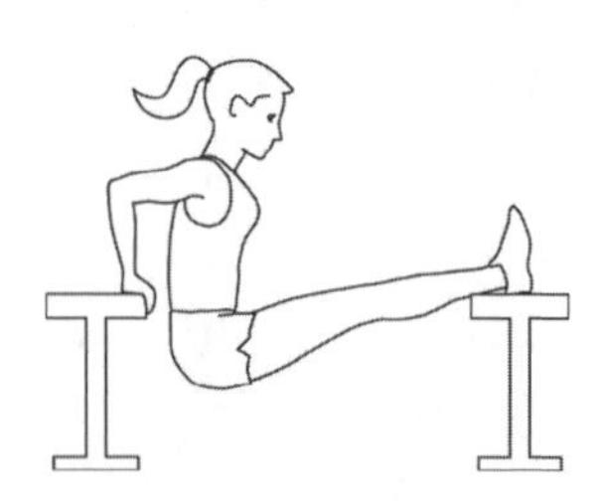

- ✳ Place a chair 3 to 5 feet from a flat stable bench (distance depends on your height).
- ✳ Make sure that the chair is solidly secured.
- ✳ With your back perpendicular to the bench, squat down and place your palms on the edge of the bench facing away from your body.
- ✳ Position you hands on the bench approximately shoulder-width apart.
- ✳ Place the heel of one foot on the chair with leg straight.
- ✳ Lift the heel of the other foot onto the chair with leg straight.
- ✳ Slowly lower your body toward the floor by bending at the elbows.
- ✳ Inhale during the lowering phase.
- ✳ Use your triceps to push your body upward to starting position.
- ✳ Exhale during the upward movement phase.

LEGS

Leg Press (Machine)

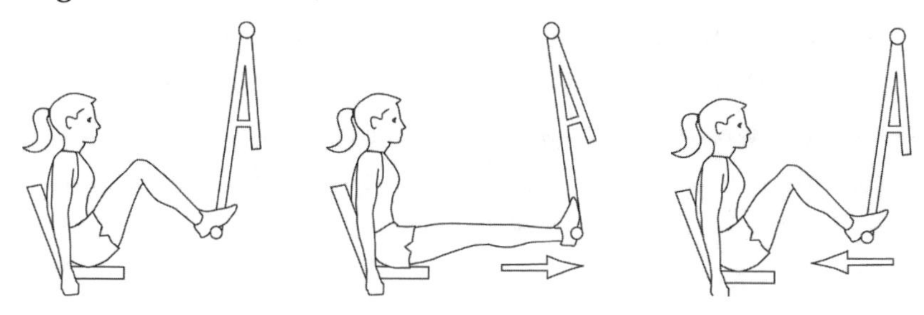

- ✳ Assume aseated position on the machine.
- ✳ Place feet shoulder-width apart in a comfortable position on the floor plate (or pedals).
- ✳ Keep your back flat against the pad and hold the hand grips.
- ✳ Push plate forward just short of locking your knees.
- ✳ Bring weight down by withdrawing your thighs to a position near your chest.

* The angle between your thigh and calf should be about 90 degrees.
* Do not bounce at bottom position.
* Inhale while lowering weight; exhale while pushing weight forward.

Leg Extension (Machine)

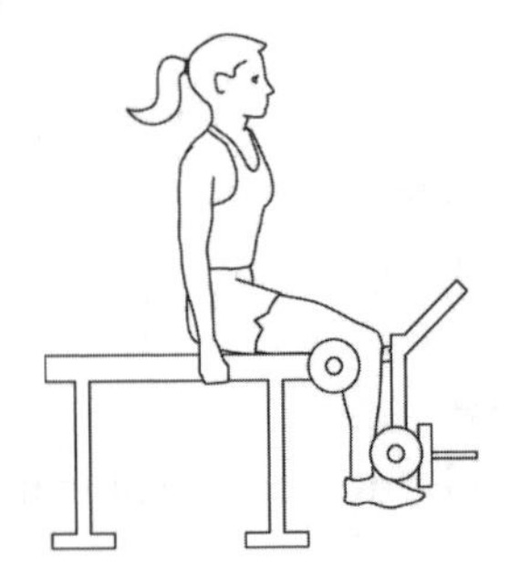
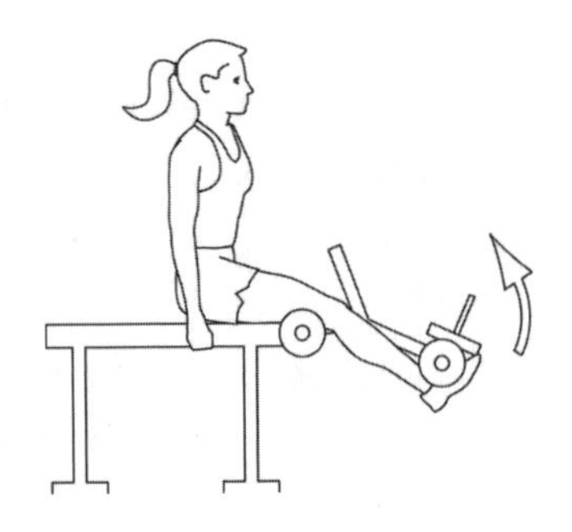

* Sit on machine with knees extended slightly over end of the seat.
* Place feet under lower foot pads.
* Grasp handles (if available) or sides of seat pad.
* Keep buttocks down and back flat against pad.
* Simultaneously extend both legs to full extension.
* Slowly return foot pad to starting position.
* Exhale through sticking point of upward movement phase; inhale during downward phase.

Leg Curl (Machine)

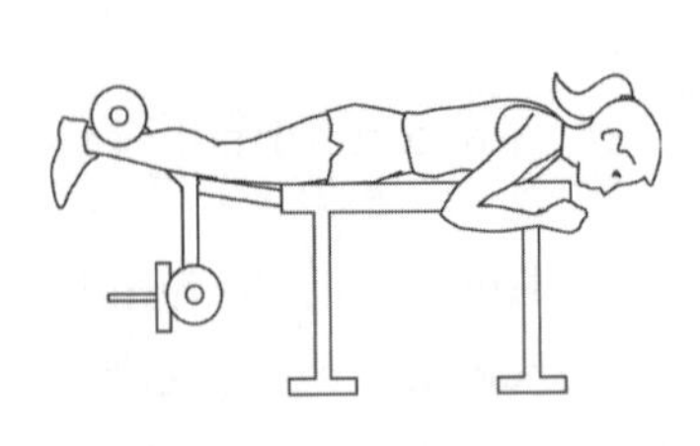
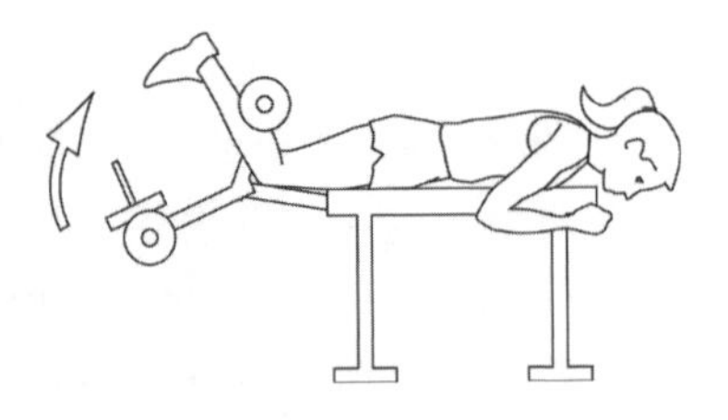

* Lie face down on the bench
* Position knees below edge of thigh pad

- ✳ Place heels under foot pad and align knees with axis of the machine.
- ✳ Grasp side handles or sides of bench pad.
- ✳ Keep hips in contact with bench.
- ✳ Flex at the knees and slowly curl the weight upward.
- ✳ Pull heels as close to the buttocks as possible.
- ✳ Slowly lower weight to full leg extension.
- ✳ Exhale during upward movement phase; inhale during downward movement phase.

  Note: Curls can be done one leg at a time or both legs at one time. Curls can also be performed in a seated leg curl machine.

Lunge (Free Weights)

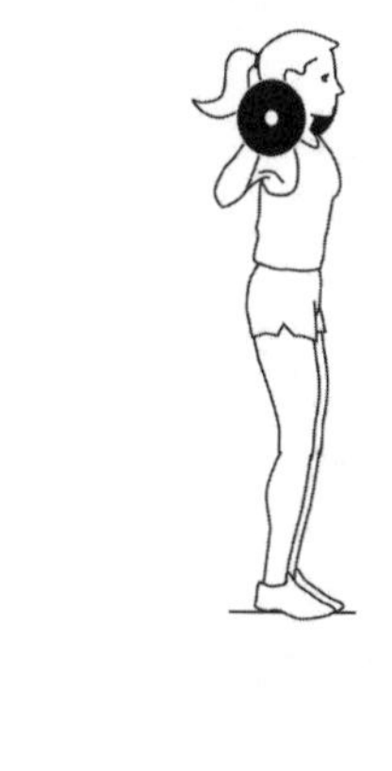

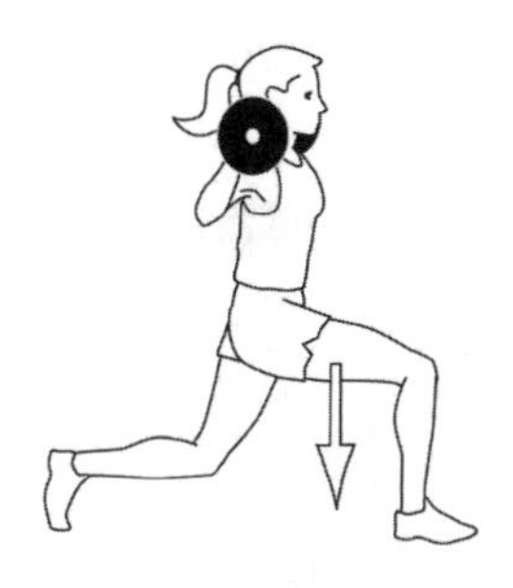

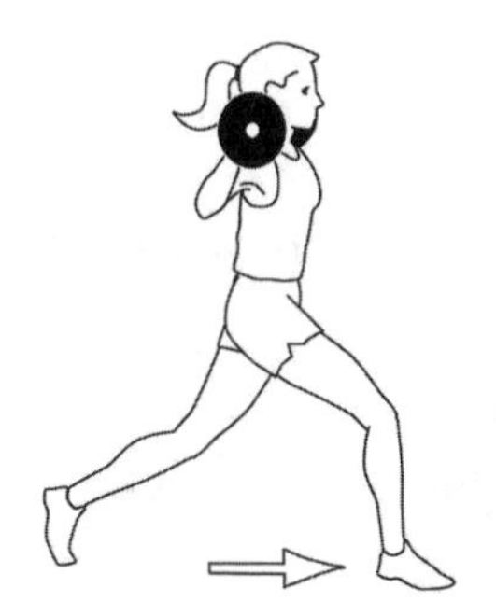

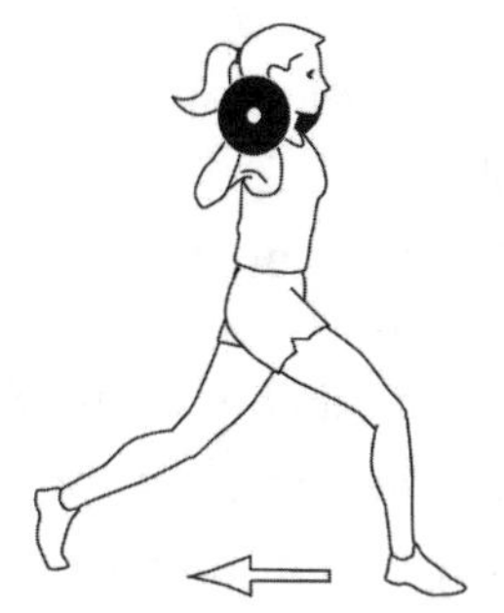

- ✳ Hold a light dumbbell in each hand.
- ✳ Take an exaggerated step forward with one leg.

- Plant lead foot squarely on floor with toes pointing straight ahead.
- Flex the lead knee slowly and under control.
- Continue flex until lead knee is directly over lead foot and thigh is parallel to the floor.
- Pause, do not bounce in the bottom position.
- Forcefully push off with lead leg.
- Return lead foot to original starting position.
- Repeat with opposite leg.
- Inhale during forward movement phase; exhale during push-off of backward movement phase.

  Note: You can also perform the lunge movement when walking forward (point A to point B) Beginners can perform the lunge using their body weight only.

Back Squat (Machine-Assisted Free Weights)

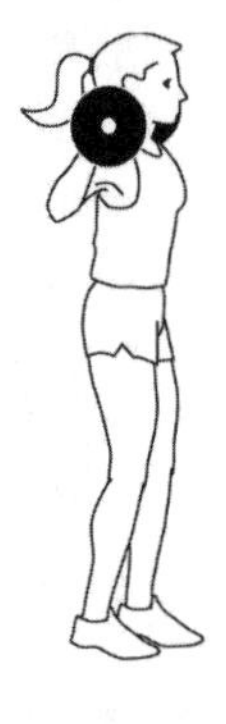

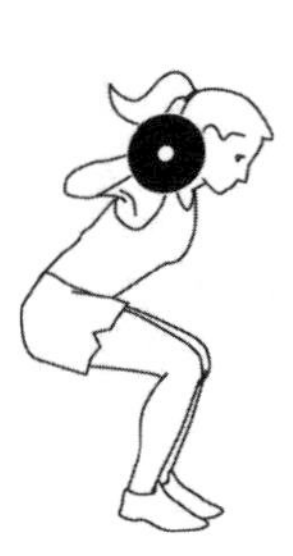

- Position the bar on the rack at approximately mid-chest height.
- Grasp the bar using an overhand grip with hands slightly wider than shoulder-width apart.
- Step under the bar with both feet.
- Place the center of the bar across your upper back.
- Elbows point toward rear.
- Hold your chest up and out.
- Straighten both legs to lift the bar off of the rack; take one or two steps back.

- ✳ Position feet shoulder-width apart with toes pointed out slightly.
- ✳ Keep feet flat on floor during exercise.
- ✳ Bend at the knees.
- ✳ Keep the weight over the middle of the foot, not over the toes.
- ✳ Descend slowly until thighs are parallel to the floor.
- ✳ Keep your back straight and head up.
- ✳ Inhale during the downward movement.
- ✳ Return to a standing position in a controlled manner.
- ✳ Keep back vertical and eyes focused ahead.
- ✳ Exhale during upward movement.
- ✳ Return barbell to rack by taking small steps with both feet.

Note: Two spotters required for this exercise.

Step-Up (Free Weights)

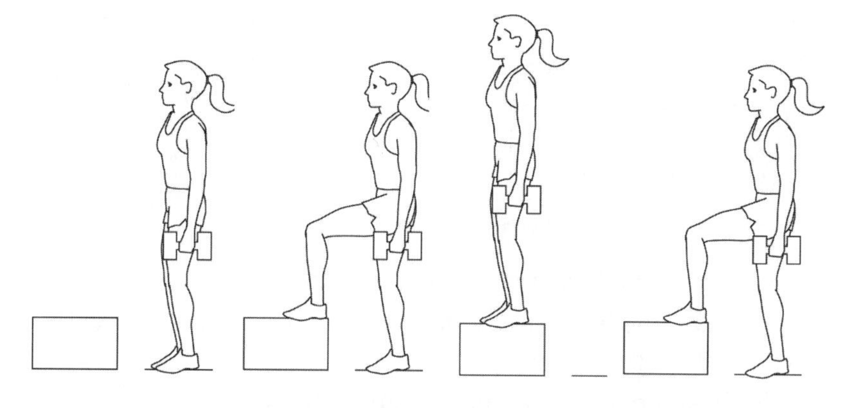

- ✳ Position in front of a step bench with arms extended down and holding a light dumbbell in each hand.
- ✳ Maintain an erect body position.
- ✳ Step with lead leg onto top of box.
- ✳ Place entire foot on center of box with toes pointing straight ahead.
- ✳ Shift body weight forward to lead leg.
- ✳ Push upward off of lead leg to a standing position on top of box.

- ✳ Do not push off with trailing leg/foot.
- ✳ Exhale during upward movement.
- ✳ At top position you should be standing straight with feet together and body weight evenly distributed.
- ✳ Step backward off of the box with original trailing leg.
- ✳ Maintain erect body position.
- ✳ Step off box with lead leg.
- ✳ Inhale during downward movement.
- ✳ Repeat step-up with other leg as lead leg.

Note: Beginners can perform step-up using body weight only (no dumbbells).

Seated Heel Raise (Machine)

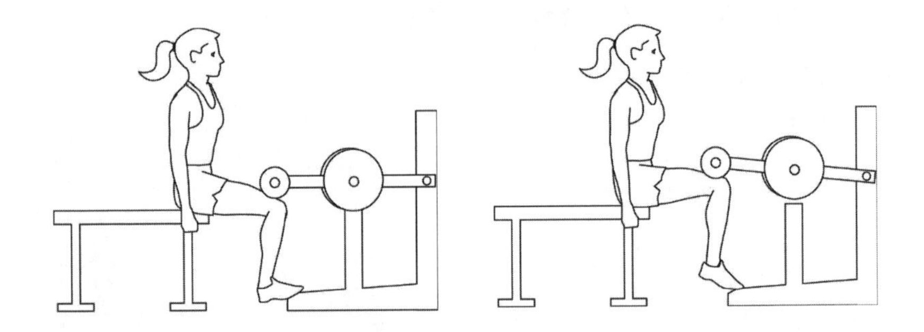

- ✳ Sit on the bench of a seated calf machine.
- ✳ Place the balls of your feet on the raised surface and close to the edge.
- ✳ Position knees under the knee pad.
- ✳ Raise your heels as high as possible, using your calf muscles to raise the knee pad.
- ✳ Pause at the top of the movement.
- ✳ Lower your heels as far as possible.
- ✳ Perform the exercise in a smooth, fluid and controlled movement.
- ✳ Exhale during upward movement, inhale during downward movement.

Standing Heel Raise (Free Weights)

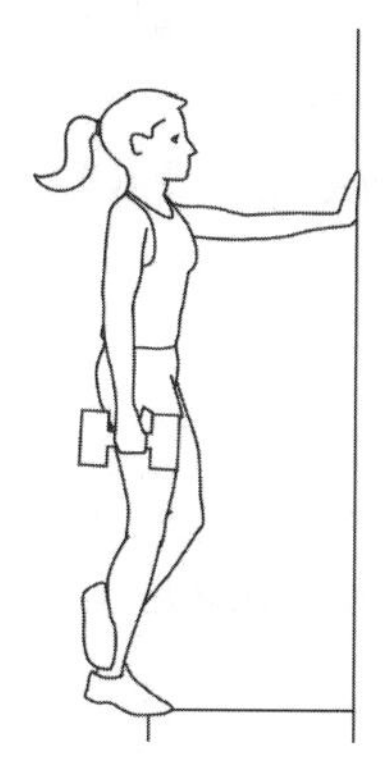

- ✳ Stand holding a barbell in your left hand with arm extended down to side.
- ✳ Step onto a slightly raised surface with your left foot.
- ✳ Raise your left heel in a slow and controlled manner as high as possible.
- ✳ Exhale during upward movement.
- ✳ Lower your left heel as far as possible.
- ✳ Inhale during downward movement.
- ✳ Repeat the exercise with right foot while holding dumbbell in your right hand.

ABDOMINALS

Abdominal exercises can be performed in multiple sets of 20 to 30 reps or in multiple 30-second intervals.

Bent-Knee Sit-Ups

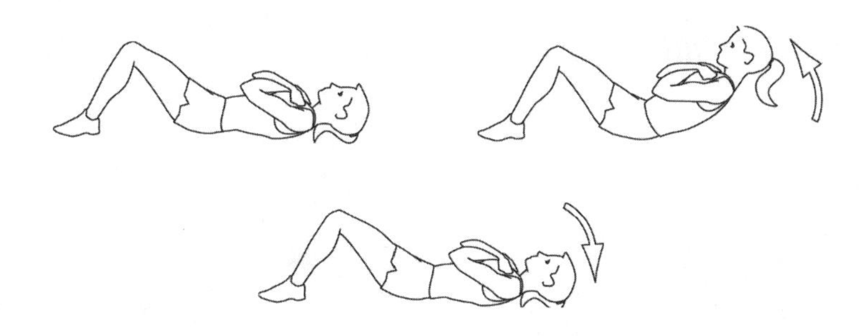

- ✳ Lie face up on a mat.
- ✳ Flex knees and bring heels close to buttocks.
- ✳ Fold arms across chest.
- ✳ Raise upper body toward thighs until upper back is off of mat.
- ✳ Keep feet flat on floor.
- ✳ Slowly return to starting position and repeat.
- ✳ Do not bounce or jerk body.
- ✳ Exhale during upward movement; inhale during downward movement.

Crunches

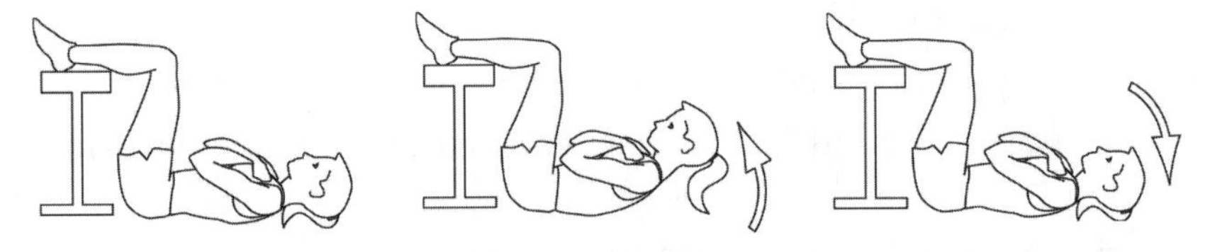

- ✳ Lie flat on back with calves and ankles resting on a bench.
- ✳ Thighs should be perpendicular to floor, lower legs (calves) parallel to floor.
- ✳ Fold arms and tuck chin to chest.
- ✳ Curl upper body forward until upper back is off of floor.
- ✳ Keep calves and ankles on bench.
- ✳ Lower shoulders slowly to floor.
- ✳ Do not bounce or jerk.
- ✳ Exhale during upward curl movement, inhale during downward movement phase.

Incline Leg Pull-in

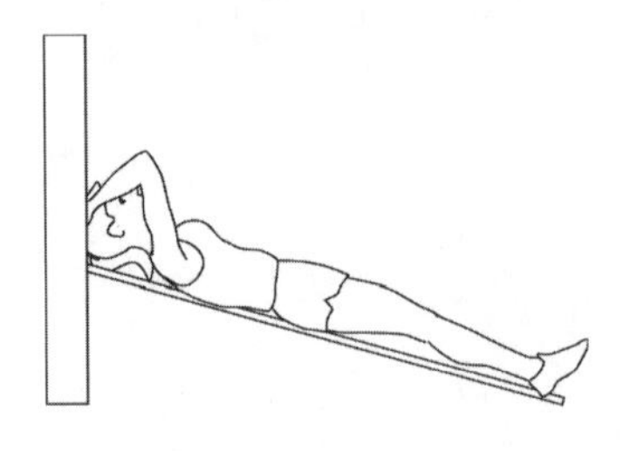

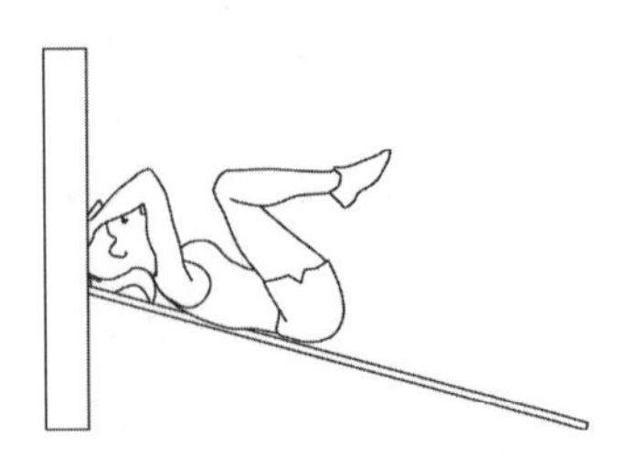

* Position a sit-up board at a 30- to 35-degree angle to the floor.
* Hold the foot bar (behind your head) with both hands.
* Flex knees and pull upper thighs into your midsection.
* Slowly return to starting position and repeat.
* Do not let your heels touch the board once you have begun the exercise.

Note: To increase resistance hold a light dumbbell between your feet during exercise.

Hip Ups

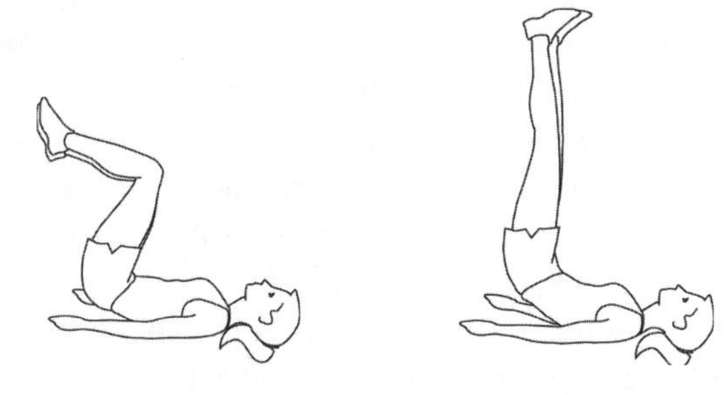

* Lie on your back with hips slightly elevated off of the floor.
* Position legs straight up in the air.
* Place hands and arms out to the side for stability.
* Raise your hips off of the ground and point toes upward.
* Pause at highest point, then slowly lower hips to ground and repeat.

Getting F.I.T. 15

Three exercise factors — **Frequency, Intensity** and **Time** (duration) — play key roles in the development of cardiovascular (aerobic) fitness. Studies show that similar gains can result from a shorter-duration high-intensity program and a longer-duration lower-intensity program. The most critical factor is matching the optimal threshold for duration with the appropriate exercise intensity. The following guidelines apply to most people. Keep in mind that you should adjust your program periodically to accommodate an improving level of fitness.

Frequency. Three workouts per week is considered to be the minimum number required to improve aerobic fitness.Exercising more often can provide additional benefits, particularly if your goal is to burn calories and lose body fat.

Intensity. How hard you exercise affects the amount of oxygen consumed and energy requirements of the activity. Monitoring your heart rate is a convenient means of estimating exercise intensity. The minimum intensity required to stimulate improvements in aerobic fitness is about 60 percent of maximum heart rate (HRmax). This value is commonly referred to as the *aerobic threshold.*

Time. Twenty to 30 minutes per workout appears to be the minimum, although a few studies conducted with very low fit individuals have demonstrated gains with as little as 10 to 15 minutes. The American College of Sports Medicine recommends 20 to 60 minutes of continuous activity per exercise session. *Note: Duration of exercise can also be prescribed in terms of distance covered or calories burned.*

Targeting the Muscles

It is a common misconception that aerobic exercise benefits only our heart and circulatory system. In actual fact our muscles benefit as well. Regular aerobic exercise improves the muscles ability to produce energy and utilize oxygen by 1) increasing the size and number of mitochondria, the miniature cellular powerhouses that produce energy aerobically; 2) increasing the concentration of aerobic enzymes needed for the breakdown of fats and carbohydrates; 3) increasing the size of muscle fibers used in training; and 4) increasing the number of capillaries serving the muscle fibers. The effect on muscles is very specific. Only those muscle fibers directly linked to the exercise are recruited for action, so improvements in aerobic fitness stimulated by one form of exercise won't necessarily transfer in totality to another form of exercise. In practical terms this means that, to produce maximum results, the biker should bike and the runner should run.

Aerobic Training Programs

Aerobic training can be subdivided into three overlapping components. *Low intensity training* is commonly referred to as *LSD* (long-slow-distance). With LSD the quantity *(volume)* of exercise takes precedent over the quality *(intensity)* of exercise. Heart rate seldom gets above 160 bpm. If your primary goal is to burn calories and lose weight, this is the program for you. *High intensity training* requires greater effort but is of shorter duration. The training heart rate range lies between 75 percent and 90 percent of HRmax. High intensity aerobic raining also improves leg strength, leg speed, and muscular endurance. *Recovery training* is lower intensity exercise typically performed on the days between harder workouts. Mean heart rate should remain at or below 130 beats per minute during recover training.

The Aerobic Training Zone

We've discussed how the minimum exercise intensity required to stimulate improvement in aerobic fitness is roughly 60 percent of HRmax. There is also an upper level of intensity, referred to as the *anaerobic (lactate) threshold,* beyond which the contribution to aerobic fitness diminishes. The upper boundary coincides with an

The Importance of Cool Down

Abrupt cessation of vigorous aerobic exercise can potentially cause pooling of blood in the lower body, circulatory problems, and next-day muscle soreness and cramps. Cool down activities (light aerobics, stretching, etc.) performed at the conclusion of a hard workout will allow your physiological systems to gradually return to their normal state of homeostasis.

exercise intensity of approximately 90 percent HRmax. An exercise heart rate falling between the lower and upper thresholds is considered to be your target training zone. You can determine your training heart rate range by performing the following steps:

Step #1. Estimate HRmax using one of the following methods:

Method 1: **The "220 – age" formula** provides a low estimate of HRmax. Using this formula a 45-year old woman would have an estimated HRmax of: *220 - 45 = 175 beats per minute (bpm)*

Method 2: **The "210 – (0.5 X age)" formula** provides a high estimate of HRmax. Using this formula a 45-year old woman would have an estimated HRmax of : *210 - (0.5 X 45) = 210- 22.5 = 187.5 bpm.* (Variability is defined by a statistic called the standard deviation [SD]). The standard deviation unit for both HRmax estimates is 12 beats per minute. This means that approximately 70 percent of all scores fall within a range of 12 beats above and 12 beats below the predicted HRmax.)

Step #2. Determine training heart rate range using one of the following methods:

Method 1: **Straight Percentage of HRmax**. Multiply HRmax by 0.6 to get the lower boundary of your aerobic training zone. Multiply by 0.9 to get the upper boundary. For example, assume that your predicted HRmax is 190 bpm. Using this method the lower threshold of your training heart rate zone is *114 bpm (0.6 X 190).* The upper threshold is *171 bpm (0.9 X 190 bpm).* Taking a straight percentage of maximal heart rate can underestimates training heart rate by approximately 15 percent.

Method 2: **The Karvonen Concept of Maximal Heart Rate Reserve.** Using this method, *training heart rate (THR) = [exercise intensity X (HRmax - HRrest)] + HRrest* where exercise intensity is the percentage of maximal intensity. Maximal heart rate reserve is defined as the difference between HRmax and resting heart rate (HRrest). Use intensities of 60 percent (0.6) and 90 percent (0.9) respectively to determine the lower and upper boundaries of your THR zone. For example, the training heart rate range for a 30-year old woman with a resting heart rate of 75 beats per minute and a HRmax of 190 beats per minute is: *Lower Boundary: THR60% = .60*

The Athlete's Heart

Studies of elite endurance athletes suggest that the heart muscle can increase in both weight and size in response to high intensity aerobic training. This condition, commonly referred to as the *athlete's heart*, was originally considered to be dangerous based on the assumption that a larger heart meant a less efficient heart. Today we know that is not the case. Increased heart size in response to regular aerobic exercise is considered a natural consequence of training that actually improves the heart's ability to perform its all important function.

X (190bpm - 75 bpm) + 75 bpm = .60 X (115) + 75 = 69 + 75 = 144 bpm; Upper boundary: THR90% = .90 X (115bpm) + 75 bpm = 103.5 + 75 = 178 bpm.

The Karvonen method provides a more accurate estimate of training heart rate than the straight percentage method, but is also more cumbersome and time consuming to calculate. The straight percentage method will suffice for most healthy adults. The slight loss in accuracy is more than compensated for by the ease of calculation.

Monitoring Heart Rate

It is easy to monitor heart rate during workouts. Stop exercising for a moment and locate your pulse by resting the index and

How to Avoid Plateaus

Most of us tend to get into an all-too-familiar exercise routine. For reasons of convenience we perform the same exercises or use the same machines for each and every workout. After a few weeks of the same old stuff our bodies adapt to those conditions. Muscles become more efficient at performing the exercise and as a result don't have to work as hard. We burn fewer calories for the same volume of exercise, and improvements in fitness begin to level off. To avoid plateaus you must constantly shock your physiological systems. You can do this by changing your exercise rotation or the types of exercises performed every few weeks. Alternate between two or three different types of aerobic exercise. Vary the duration and intensity of your workouts as well.

middle finger at the base of the wrist, or at the side of the neck near to your Adam's apple. Count the beats for 15 seconds and then multiply by four. Your exercise heart rate should fall somewhere between the lower and upper boundaries of your target training zone. After a while you will be able to judge whether you are "in the zone" simply by gauging how you feel. Cues such as sweating, breathing patterns, and aching muscles will help to gauge exercise intensity.

Evaluating Progress

A written log will allow you to step back in time and compare where you are today with where you were then. Make note of the frequency, intensity and duration of your aerobic workouts. Record changes in body weight and body measurements. With that in mind never lose sight of the fact that you can't gauge progress solely based on the number of pounds lost. Improvements in how you feel, physically as well as emotionally, are equally if not more important.

Rating the Aerobic Exercises 16

The key to reaping the many benefits that aerobic exercise has to offer can be summed up in one word — consistency. It is not so much a function of the type of activity you choose but rather how often you do it. With that in mind, the best exercise for you personally is the one (or more) that you are willing to do on a regular basis. You have a wide variety of choices. Depending on your fitness goals, some may provide more benefits than others.

Walking

Benefits. Our most popular aerobic exercise with more than 90 million participants. Walking is low impact, easy on the joints, and the risk of injury is minimal. No special skills are required, and workouts can be done virtually anywhere it is safe to walk. A good pair of walking shoes is really all you need to get started.

Energy Burn. Moderate. Walking one mile will burn approximately the same number of calories (60 to 100 depending upon body weight) as jogging a mile. It will just take you longer to do it. It usually takes 1800 to 2200 walking steps to equal one mile, depending upon stride length.

Limitations. It takes longer to realize cardiovascular benefits than with more intense forms of aerobic exercise. Walking does little to condition the upper body.

Jogging

Benefits. Jogging is a versatile form of exercise that can be adapted to a variety of fitness levels. There is a low to moderate risk of injury that increases slightly as daily and weekly mileage goes up.

Energy Burn. Moderate-high to high.

Limitations. Jogging may be too strenuous for severely overweight individuals or those with arthritic joints. It does little to condition the upper body.

Race Walking

Benefits. Provides basically all of the benefits of jogging but places less stress on the ankles and knees. The primary differences between race walking and regular walking deal with form and intensity. Proper race walking form requires that the toe of one foot remain on the ground until the heel of the opposite foot touches. The exaggerated arm swing burns additional calories and provides a limited upper body workout as well. At its most competitive extreme, race walking can be a full-fledged endurance event.

Energy Burn. Moderate to high. You can increase the intensity of workouts by including hills in your walking course. Hill walking burns up to 25 percent more calories than walking on a level surface.

Limitations. The walking motion may seem awkward until you get used to it.

Outdoor Bicycling

Benefits. Easy on the joints and has a low incidence of injury (unless you crash!). Biking can provide an excellent cardiovascular workout when peddling over varied terrain.

Energy Burn. Moderate. The calorie burn is similar to brisk walking, and will vary depending upon body size and exercise intensity.

Limitations. Biking outdoors can be risky depending upon the local traffic situation. Workouts do little to condition the upper body.

Stationary Bicycling

Benefits. Low impact and easy on the joints. Doesn't require the balance and coordination of outdoor biking. You will never have to cancel your workout because of poor weather. Very low risk of injury.

Energy Burn. Moderate.

Limitations. Does not provide much of an upper body workout, although some bikes require you to use a pumping action of the arms while pedaling.

Treadmill

Benefits. Similar to walking and jogging, depending upon the intensity of your workout. Fairly low impact and easy on the joints. Motorized treadmills make it easy for you to adjust exercise intensity.

Energy Burn. Moderate.

Limitations. The initial cost can be substantial so it is important to invest wisely. A motorized treadmill is preferred over a non-motorized unit. A quality machine will generally fall in the $2000 to $4000 price range.

Jumping Rope

Benefits. Minimal amount of equipment (rope and well-cushioned shoes) can be easily packed and carried with you when traveling. You can workout almost anywhere - indoors, outdoors, at home, or in a hotel room.

Energy Burn.Moderate-high to high.

Limitations. Harder on the joints than walking or cycling. High intensity rope jumping requires a fair amount of coordination.

Stair Climber Machine

Benefits. An excellent choice for improving cardiovascular fitness, body composition, and lower body strength and endurance. Workouts on a machine are lower impact and less stressful than running up and down actual stairs. There is also less chance of injury.

Energy Burn. Moderate-high to high.

Limitations. Stair climbing may be too strenuous for people who are greatly overweight. Workouts do little to condition your upper body. A quality machine costs between $2500 and $4000. Cheaper models are available, but you will usually get what you pay for.

Elliptical Trainer

Benefits. Combines the best of running and stair climbing. Smooth exercise motion is easy on the joints. Most machines have handle bars that move back and forth, so you get a limited upper body workout as well.

Energy Burn. Comparable to jogging.

Limitations. Coordinating movement of arms and legs may feel awkward for beginning exercisers.

Swimming

Benefits. Swimming is a great exercise for improving cardiovascular fitness, muscular endurance, and body composition. An excellent choice for people with joint or arthritic conditions.

Energy Burn. Moderate to high.

Limitations. Swimming requires a higher level of skill than most forms of aerobic exercise. Convenience can also be a problem as you will need access to a pool or body of water. Speaking from personal experience, if you are not a good swimmer it's not much fun!

Rowing

Benefits. Rowing can provide a low-impact, total body workout that is easy on the joints and has a low injury rate. It is a great alternative to biking and running provided you know the proper technique. Vigorous rowing stresses the cardiovascular system while also working muscles in the abdomen, back, arms and legs. Workouts can be performed indoors (rowing machines) or in the natural setting.

Energy Burn. High.

Limitations. Outdoor rowing requires access to a body of water or river and a certain degree of skill. Equipment (canoe, paddles, and life jackets) is more costly than that required for most other forms of aerobic exercise.

Cross Country (Nordic) Skiing

Benefits. The ultimate aerobic exercise. Cross-country skiing will develop cardiovascular fitness, improve body composition, and burn tremendous amounts of energy. It is easy on the joints and has a low injury rate.

Energy Burn. Very high.

Limitations. Outdoor skiing is possible only in certain areas of the country and during certain seasons of the year. Equipment can be somewhat costly, although not nearly so expensive as most exercise machines. The simulated skiing motion of indoor ski machines may feel awkward to beginners.

Hiking/Backpacking

Benefits. Great way to spend a day outdoors. Hiking over hilly terrain provides an excellent lower body workout. If you are carrying and balancing a pack it can provide an upper body workout as well. Hiking burns more calories than normal walking and is relatively easy on the joints.

Energy Burn. High to very high.

Limitations. Convenience can be a problem if you live in an urban area.

Aerobic Dance

Benefits. Dance away the pounds. Workouts can be performed at home (video) or in a social setting. Vigorous aerobic dancing can strengthen muscles and improve cardiovascular fitness.

Energy Burn. Moderate to high.

Limitations. High impact aerobic dance can be stressful to joints and muscles. Low-impact may not be vigorous enough to push your heart rate into the training zone

Roller Skating/Blading

Benefits. It is relatively easy on the joints if you don't fall too often! Vigorous skating can provide a total body workout.

Energy Burn. Moderate-high to high

Limitations. Requires more equipment (skates, knee guards, helmet) than walking or jogging. Risk of injury is greater than with most other types of aerobic exercise.

Improving Flexibility 17

As we get older all of us should make an effort to maintain and, if need be, improve our range-of-motion. Although flexibility exercises do not require any special skills or expertise, it is important to perform stretches correctly. Static stretches that utilize a slow and steady extension of the targeted muscles are preferred over ballistic (bouncing) movements. Perform each stretch in two stages.

Stage #1: The Easy Stretch. Ease into the stretch by slowly extending the target muscle or muscle group until you feel tightness. Maintain the stretch position for 15 to 30 seconds, then relax for a moment before moving into the second stage.

Stage #2: The Developmental Stretch. Slowly move into a deeper stretch. A feeling of tension in the target muscle is a signal to stop and hold the stretch. Do not stretch to the point of pain. Hold the stretch position for 15 to 30 seconds.

When to Stretch

Include stretching exercises in your pre-workout warm-up and post-workout cool-down. In some instances you can include stretching exercises within your workouts; for example, while resting between multiple sets of strength-training exercises. Stretching immediately after exercise may actually be more beneficial for improving range-of-motion than pre-exercise stretching.

Stretching Do's and Don'ts

To ensure that your stretching program is both safe and effective adhere to the following guidelines ...

- Never stretch a cold muscle. Warm-up with several minutes of light aerobic exercise prior to stretching.
- Isolate the muscle or group of muscles being stretched.
- Ease slowly into each stretch to prevent activation of the stretch reflex.
- Breathe normally with emphasis on the exhalation when moving into the deeper stretch. Do not hold your breath.

Stretching Should Never Be a Competition

Individuals may vary greatly in their degree of flexibility. For that reason stretching should never be viewed as a competition among friends. Measure progress against your own standards and initial state of flexibility. The primary goal is to improve range-of-motion in a safe, injury-free manner — not to outstretch your training partner.

- Extend the stretch until you feel tightness (but not pain) in the muscle. Hold the stretch position for 15 to 30 seconds, and then slowly ease out of the stretch.
- Perform each stretch twice; move into a deeper stretch the second time around.
- When stretching with a partner make sure to communicate with one another; do not force your partner into a deeper stretch than she or he is capable of achieving.

Stretch Exercises

Perform stretching exercises five or more days per week. Choose at least one exercise for each category listed below.

HAMSTRINGS

Straight Leg Sitting Hamstring Stretch

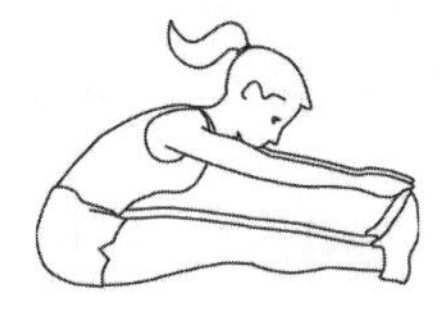
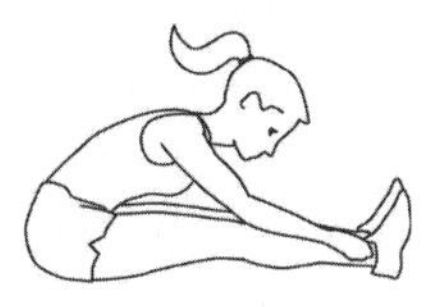
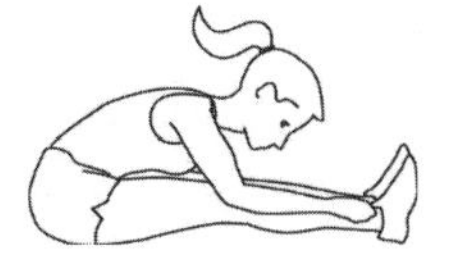

- Sit on the floor with legs extended.
- Keep legs straight and together.
- Lean forward with arms extended and attempt to touch your toes.

Hurdlers Hamstring Stretch

- Assume a sitting position with your right leg straight and left leg bent 90 degrees.

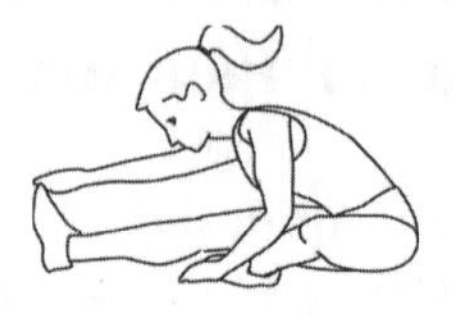 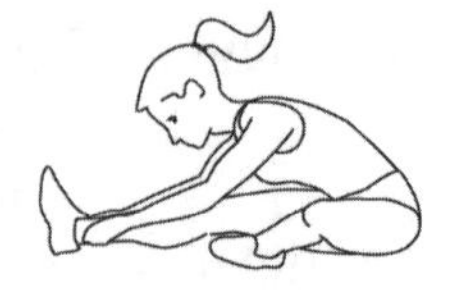 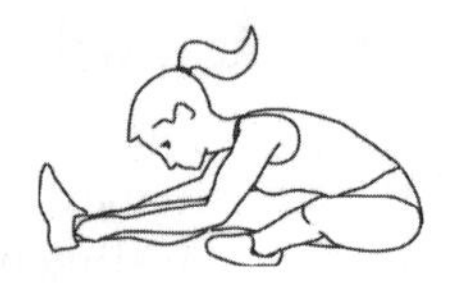

* Position the heel of your left foot against the inside of your right thigh.
* Bend forward at the waist and attempt to touch your right foot with both hands. Keep your right leg straight.
* Repeat stretch with opposite leg.

Split Leg Stretch

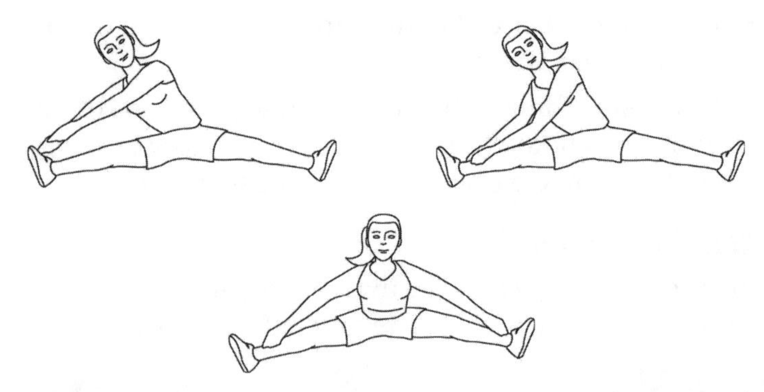

* Assume a sitting position with legs spread at a 45-degree angle.
* Keep your knees locked and legs tight to the floor.
* Lower your head as far as possible toward your right knee and hold that position.
* Keep your back straight and abdominal muscles tight during the stretch.
* Repeat the stretch toward your left knee.

QUADRICEPS (THIGH)

Forward Lunge Stretch

* Begin in a standing position.
* Step forward with your right leg. Flex the knee at a 90-degree angle. At this point the thigh of your right leg should be parallel to floor.

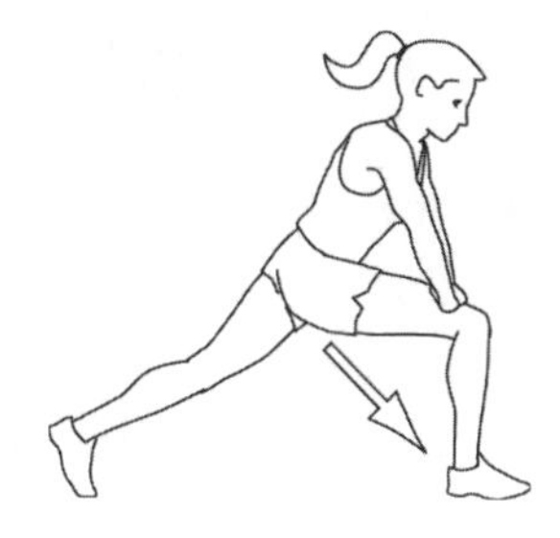

- ✳ Place both hands on your right thigh for support.
- ✳ Extend your left leg back with heel off of the floor.
- ✳ Repeat the stretch with left leg bent and right leg extended back.

Lying on Stomach Quad Stretch

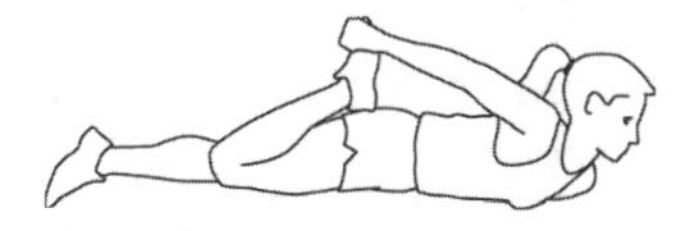

- ✳ Lie on stomach with legs extended behind.
- ✳ Flex one leg at the knee and bring the heel towards your buttocks.
- ✳ Reach behind and grasp the ankle. Slowly pull the heel closer to your buttocks until you feel tightness in the thigh.
- ✳ Repeat stretch with the opposite leg.

Standing Quad Stretch

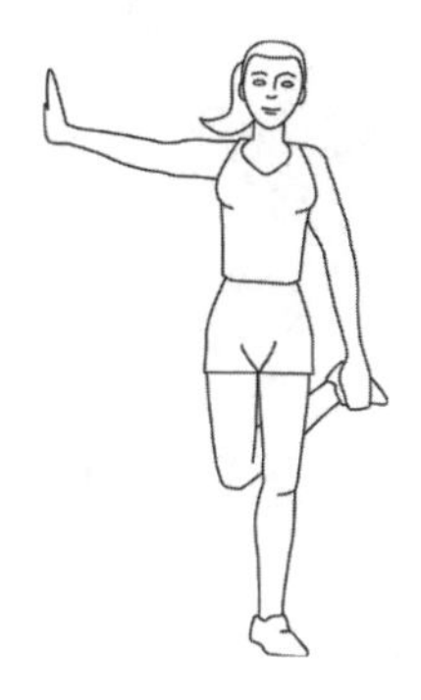

- ✳ Stand facing a wall at arms length

- Lean forward and use your right arm to brace yourself against the wall.
- Flex your right leg at the knee.
- Reach behind with the left arm and grasp the right ankle.
- Pull the heel of the right foot closer to your buttock, until you feel tightness in the upper thigh area.
- Repeat the stretch with your opposite leg.

Side Quad Stretch

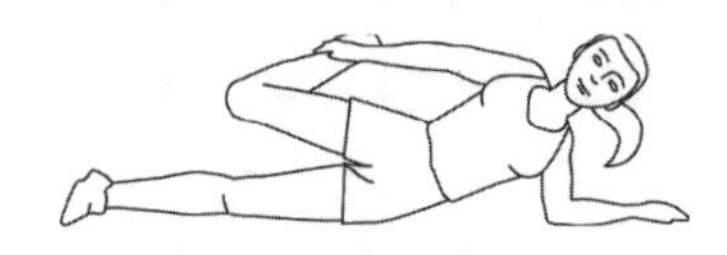

- Lie on your left side.
- Place your left forearm flat on floor with upper arm perpendicular to the floor.
- Flex your right leg, grasp right ankle with right hand and pull it towards buttocks.
- Move the knee backward and slightly upward as you stretch.
- Repeat stretch with opposite leg.

GROIN

Sitting Groin Stretch (Butterfly)

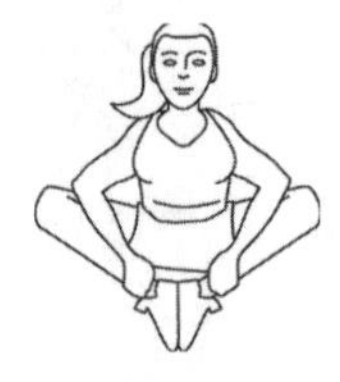

- Assume a sitting position with the soles of your feet pressed together in front.
- Grasp your feet with both hands, and position your elbows on the inside surface of your knees.
- Use the elbows to gently push your knees downward.

Lying Groin Stretch

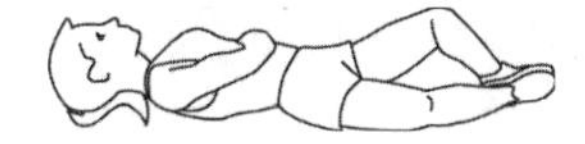

- ✳ Lie flat on your back.
- ✳ Flex your knees at approximately 90 degrees.
- ✳ Press the soles of your feet together in front.
- ✳ Spread your legs sideways.
- ✳ Lower the outside surface of each knee as close to the ground as possible.

LOWER BACK

Standing Lower Back Stretch

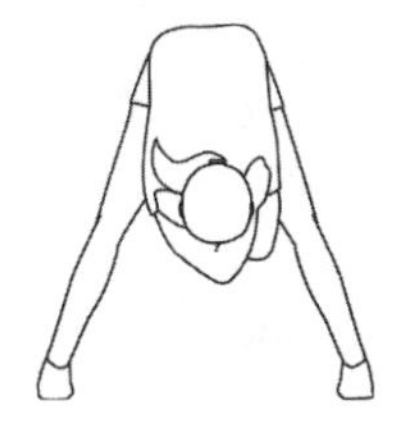

- ✳ Stand with feet spread shoulder-width apart and knees slightly flexed.
- ✳ Cross your arms, bend forward at the waist, and lower one elbow as close to the floor as possible.
- ✳ Return to upright position and repeat the stretch with the opposite elbow.

Lying Back Stretch

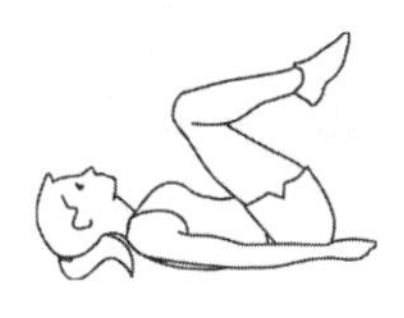

- ✳ Lie on your back with arms extended to the sides and palms facing downward.

* Slowly bring your knees up toward your chin as far as possible without raising your arms and hands off of the floor.
* Lift your hips slightly off of floor.

Spinal Twist

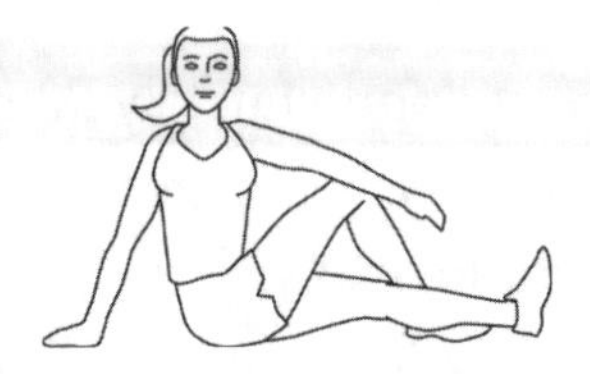

* Sit with legs straight and upper body nearly vertical.
* Place your right foot outside of the left knee.
* Place your right palm on the floor behind you.
* Push your right knee to the left with left elbow while turning your shoulders and head to the right as far as possible.
* Repeat the stretch with your left leg.

SHOULDERS

Behind-the-Back Arm Stretch

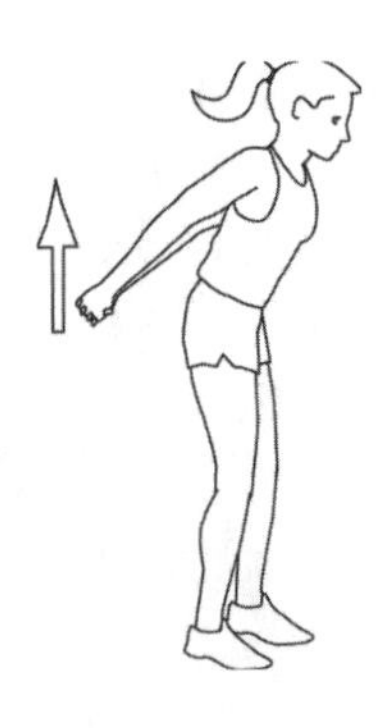

* Extend both arms behind with hands at approximately waist height.
* Interlock fingers.
* Keep arms straight and extended behind as you gradually raise them as far as possible.

Behind-the-Head Elbow Pull

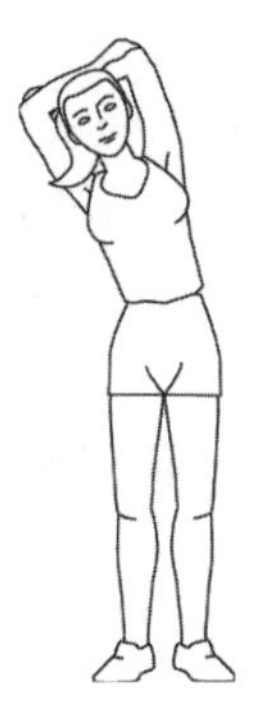

- ✳ Place one arm behind your head with elbow bent at 90-degrees.
- ✳ Grasp the elbow with your opposite hand, and gently pull it farther behind your head.
- ✳ Hold the stretch position.
- ✳ Repeat the stretch with opposite arm positioned behind your head.

Arm-Across-Chest Pull

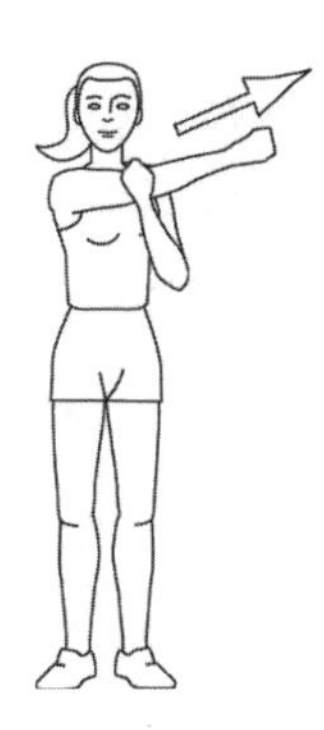

- ✳ Extend right arm across the front of your chest.
- ✳ Grasp the right elbow with your left hand and gently pull to the left.
- ✳ Repeat the stretch in the opposite direction using the right hand to pull the left arm across the chest.

NECK

Static Neck Stretch

- ✳ Place your right hand to the left side of head.
- ✳ Slowly pull head down and sideways toward the right shoulder.
- ✳ Do not jerk!
- ✳ Repeat the stretch to opposite side with your left hand.

Flexion and Extension

- ✳ Stand erect.
- ✳ Flex your neck forward by tucking the chin toward chest.
- ✳ Hold that position for 15-30 seconds.
- ✳ Relax, then extend your neck and head backward as far as is comfortably possible. Hold that position for 15-30 seconds.

Eating for Optimal Fitness 18

By Leslie Bonci, M.P.H., R.D.

Well, if you've read this far through the book, you've already made a significant investment in your fitness. What, when and how much you eat can improve or detract from your fitness. If your goal is to be as fit as you can, you will want to make sure you are feeding your body optimally. Sounds easy, right? Well actually, it should be, but unfortunately, the message given to women, even active women, is often one of restriction or exclusion when it comes to eating. Not only is this totally unfair, but this type of eating attitude will only hurt your fitness goals.

It is not cool not to eat, and it certainly detracts from your fitness levels. Agonizing over the calories or fat grams in a particular food can be mentally draining, and if this mindset results in short-changing the body when it comes to essential fuel for sport, the result is going to be a decrease in all aspects of fitness.

Let's set the record straight. There is no such thing as "perfect" when it comes to body, and even though we all know someone who we think may have the "perfect" body, that does not mean she has the "perfect" life. Is it possible to be fit and fueled? Absolutely, but sometimes we have to ignore some of the negative media messages. I want you to focus on what your body allows you to do, and how enjoyable and rewarding that is. When one of my female athletes tells me she is unhappy with her thighs or rear end, I gently remind her that those very thighs and butt allow her to walk into my office and participate in her sport. None of us walk around with our weight tattooed on our arm or forehead, or our clothing size outside of our clothes. But, isn't it amazing how many times an article about a female athlete never fails to mention if she has had weight issues. How many stories about male athletes focus on their waist circumference? Not many!

I am suggesting we focus instead on achieving a fit, fueled body. No one can see your weight, but they can see toned muscles, a healthy glow, confidence and a YES I CAN attitude. You go, girl! If this is your goal, you are going to need to pay attention to what goes into your body more than friends or family member who are not active.

If you are going to have an active lifestyle, on a competitive or recreational basis, you need to provide your body with the right amount and right kind of fuel. To perform your best, whether running on the street, cycling on a trail, or lifting at the gym, you need to be aware that food is the fuel for activity. If you haven't eaten for several hours before a workout you will have less strength, speed and stamina, and your concentration suffers as well. Instead of giving 100 percent during your workout, you'll be lucky to give 50 percent! Let's examine the role that nutrition plays in fitness.

All foods are composed of some combination of the three major nutrients: carbohydrate, protein and fat These nutrients are broken down in the body to the following substrates, some of which are used for body functions, as well as providing fuel for exercise. The following table illustrates how the body uses nutrients, and metabolites, or products of nutrient digestion.

TABLE 18.1: Nutrient Utilization and Functions

NUTRIENT	METABOLITE	FUNCTIONS
Carbohydrate	Glucose	Fuel for the brain Blood glucose can be a fuel for exercise Glucose can be stored as glycogen in the muscle and liver to be used during exercise
Protein	Amino acids	Used to maintain lean muscle mass Boosts the immune system Helps to keep bones healthy Used minimally as a fuel source for exercise
Fat	Fatty acids	Used to insulate the body Provides essential fatty acids Used as a fuel source for endurance exercise

The best eating plan for an active female includes a mix of these three nutrients throughout the day. No athlete is going to do better by cutting out carbohydrates or eating a totally fat-free diet. In addition, the food choices would be incredibly monotonous!

If you are doing an all out sprint, the body uses exclusively carbohydrate to fuel your working muscles. If you eat a diet that is too low in carbohydrates, your body does not have enough stored carbohydrate (glycogen) in reserve, and you will not be able to perform at your best. If you are doing a distance run or cycling event, playing a soccer game, or hiking all day, your body uses an equivalent amount of stored carbohydrate (glycogen) and fat as fuel sources. Protein is not a major player in terms of a fuel source for exercise. This is why you need to make sure you have enough nutrients in the meals before exercise, and especially during training so that your body has the reserves to draw on. If the gas tank is empty in your car, or your bike's tires are flat, you won't go anywhere any time soon. Same thing applies to your body. You need to fuel it to move it!

In addition to the role that food plays as a fuel substrate for exercise, you need to think about how much to eat per day. It is very important to eat enough for sport, but do be aware that the needs will vary depending upon age. We can look at daily requirements through different eating plans. Using the food guide pyramid as an example, one can determine daily needs using the pyramid as a guide.

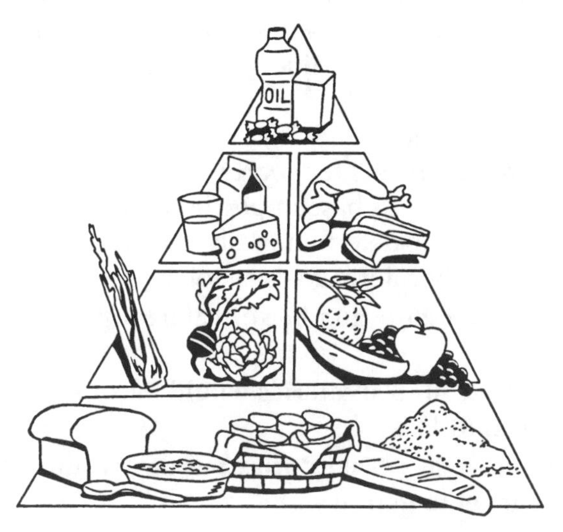

TABLE 18.2: Food Guide Pyramid Suggested Daily Servings by Calorie Needs

	CALORIE LEVEL		
	1600	2200	2800
FOOD GROUP			
Grain	6	9	11
Vegetable	3	4	5
Fruit	2	3	4
Dairy*	2-3	2-3	2-3
Meat (ounces)	5	6	7
Fat (grams)	53	73	93

Teenage girls and women who are pregnant or breastfeeding require 3 servings of dairy foods daily.

The first step would be to determine which calorie level is best for you. The guidelines are as follows:

CATEGORY	CALORIE LEVEL
Children	2200
Teens	2200
Women	1600-2800*
Older women	1600-2200*

* *The higher calories would be appropriate for a women exercising strenuously most days of the week*

Table 18.2 depicts the number of servings from the food groups for each calorie level. The goal is to include ALL of the groups daily, not to pick and choose. Eating this way helps to ensure balance and variety in your diet in addition to meeting nutritional requirements.

Another way for active adolescents and women to determine daily nutrient requirements for sport would be to calculate calorie and nutrient requirements based upon body weight. The following guide illustrates how to determine daily needs. The first step would be to determine daily calorie goals as follows:

Weight (pounds) x 20 = number of calories per day for weight maintenance

Weight (pounds) x 20 –300 calories would be an appropriate calorie level for weight loss

Weight (pounds) x 20 + 500 calories per day would be an appropriate calorie level to gain weight

The recommended composition of the diet for optimal performance is carbohydrate: 60 percent, protein: 15 percent and fat 25 percent.

In order to calculate the appropriate number of servings of carbohydrate, protein and fat–containing foods required daily, we must first determine how many grams of each of these nutrients are necessary. This calculation is done as follows:

Carbohydrate requirements in grams = .60 x daily calories divided by 4

Protein requirements in grams = .15 x daily calories divided by 4

Fat requirements in grams = .25 x daily calories divided by 9

EXAMPLE: 150 pound female athlete would need 3000 calories per day to maintain her weight: weight (pounds x 20) Her nutrient needs would be as follows: Carbohydrate needs: .60 x 3000 divided by 4 = 450 grams of carbohydrate, Protein needs: .15 x 3000 divided by 4 = 112 grams of protein, Fat needs: .25 x 3000 divided by 9 = 80 grams of fat.

To help you to select an appropriate number of food choices daily, I have provided a table listing various weights and corresponding nutrient needs. Pick the weight that most closely matches your own, or where you would like to be. For example, if you weigh 135, but would like to be 130, then use the values listed for 130 pounds as your daily guide.

Table 18.3 lists the calories, carbohydrate, protein and fat selections for different body weights. The number of selections for each nutrient were calculated as follows:

Carbohydrate food choices contain 50 grams of carbohydrate.

Protein food choices contain 20 grams of protein.

Fat containing food choices have 10 grams of fat.

To construct a diet for optimal performance, CIRCLE the choices you like from each list in Table 18-4 on the following pages and try to have a food from each category every time you eat.

I realize that the amount of food listed may be overwhelming to you. Keep in mind that these are suggested amounts. You will need to decide what is appropriate for you and make changes gradually. You may want to add one serving at a time, or even one half serving at a time, if this is more comfortable.

Now that you have figured out the right amount of food for you, the next step is how to get the most out of this food. An active body will perform best when you fuel it every few hours. I am a big

TABLE 18.3: Determining Daily Requirements

Weight	Calories	Carbohydrate selections	Protein selections	Fat selections
80	1600	5	3	4
85	1700	5	3	4.5
90	1800	5.5	3.5	5
95	1900	6	3.5	5
100	2000	6	4	5.5
105	2100	6.5	4	5.5
110	2200	7	4	6
115	2300	7	4	6.4
120	2400	7	4.5	6.5
125	2500	7.5	4.75	7
130	2600	8	5	7
135	2700	8	5	7.5
140	2800	8.5	5	8
145	2900	8.75	5.5	8
150	3000	9	5.5	8
155	3100	9	5.75	8.5
160	3200	9.5	6	9
165	3300	10	6	9
170	3400	10	6.5	9.5
175	3500	10.5	6.5	9.75
180	3600	10.75	6.75	10
185	3700	11	7	10
190	3800	11.5	7	10.5
195	3900	11.75	7.5	10.5
200	4000	12	7.5	11
205	4100	12	7.75	11.5
210	4200	12.5	8	11.5
215	4300	13	8	12
220	4400	13	8.25	12.25

believer in eating something every 3-4 hours, starting with within one hour of waking up. Not only does eating this way give you a constant fuel supply, but it can prevent overeating later in the day. A good rule of thumb with meals before exercise is as follows:

3-4 hrs before exercise	*2 hrs before*	*1 hr before*
Turkey sandwich	Cereal with milk	Sports drink
Pasta with sauce	Yogurt and cereal	Piece of fruit
Stir-fry over rice	Bagel with peanut butter	Cereal bar

The closer your meal is to exercise time, the lighter it should be. Try to limit high fat foods before exercise (fried items, fatty meats) as they can cause gastrointestinal distress. High fiber foods before exercise, such as dried fruit or bran cereals may have a laxative effect. Apple juice, caffeine-containing beverages, and high sugar drinks such as fruit punch or fruit drink can also increase the frequency of bowel movements and may not be the best choice before exercise. Again, you need to determine what foods, the amount of them, and the timing of eating that works best for you.

If you are preparing for an event, such as adventure race, a distance run, all day hike, bike race or cross country skiing, you may want to try adding more to your diet in the days leading up to your competition or activity. All of us have heard of, or even attended pasta parties the night before a race. One night of pasta will not allow the body to store enough extra fuel to make a difference in the next day's performance. If you are trying to optimize fuel storage for a better outcome, you will want to add more carbohydrate into your diet four days before your event. The easiest way to do this is to add extra carbohydrate at each meal:

A slice of toast
A piece of fruit
½ cup of cereal
½ cup of rice or pasta

Much has been written about the need to fuel the body during exercise. Some of the early studies indicated that fueling during exercise was necessary only if one is exercising longer than 90 minutes. Newer studies have shown the benefits of fuel during intense activity lasting only 30 minutes. So what should you do? You need to experiment to find out what works for you. I am a marathon runner and find that on my longer runs, I need to have sports drink in order to get through my run. It certainly isn't practical or necessary to sit down to a full course meal in the middle of a workout, but if you are at the gym working hard or playing a team sport , you may want to try refueling during breaks or in the middle of your workout. Some athletes have found that a little honey works well, others rely on sports drinks. Experiment, have fun, see what works, and when you find something you like, make sure you have it with you at all times! It is essential to get in enough fluid during your workouts or in competition. We'll discuss fluid strategies a little later.

TABLE 18.4: Food Lists

CARBOHYDRATE*

A large bagel
1-1/2 cups pasta
1 cup of rice
A cup of Cheerios
A low-fat fruit muffin
2 cups of oatmeal
1 cup of applesauce
A large baked potato
1 cup of corn
5 fig bars
1-1/2 cups of grapes
1-1/2 English muffins
4 4-inch diameter pancakes
1 cup pudding
2 handfuls of pretzels
2 cups of juice
1-1/2 cups frozen yogurt
32 oz sports drink
2 packets flavored oatmeal
25 animal crackers
2 bananas
2 cups of grapes
10 large marshmallows
Licorice, 1 2 oz package
¾ cup granola
2 cereal bars
20 jelly beans
16 oz lemonade/fruit punch
1-1/2 cups sweetened cereal
½ bag of microwave low-fat popcorn
1 Pop Tart
15 vanilla wafers
½ cup raisins

PROTEIN**

A computer mouse size:
Piece of chicken
Piece of beef
Piece of fish
A 3 oz. can of tuna
¾ cup of cottage cheese
1 soy burger
1-1/2 cups pinto beans
3 slices of cheese
3 thin slices of lunch meat
3 eggs
A mayonnaise jar lid sized:
Hamburger or turkey burger
¾ cup egg substitute
8 oz. tofu

HIGH FAT CARBOHYDRATE FOODS

Try to limit!
Not as performance boosting!
Most cookies
Chocolate
Chips
French fries
Doughnuts
Ice cream

FAT***

A tablespoon of peanut butter
¼ cup of nuts
2 pats of butter
2 tsp of mayonnaise
2 tsp of oil
2 strips of bacon
2 tablespoons cream cheese
4 tablespoons sour cream
1 tablespoon of regular salad dressing
2 tablespoons of Light salad dressing

DOUBLE DUTY FOODS:

Carbohydrate + protein

Yogurt 8 oz container=
50 g carbohydrate + 12 gs of protein
Sportsbars:(PowerBar, GatorBar, etc.)
Certain beverage supplements: Gatorade Nutrition Shake, Boost, Carnation Instant Breakfast
Milk: 16 ounces chocolate milk = 50 grams carbohydrate, 16 grams protein
Cheese pizza (2 slices = 80 grams of carbohydrate, 16 grams of protein!)

* There are many nutrition myths surrounding the use of carbohydrate-containing foods. Some people believe these foods are fattening and will cause weight gain, while other believe that they can be addicted to carbohydrates. These foods are essential for optimal fitness. You can be selective about the types of carbohydrate foods you choose, leaning toward whole grain breads and cereals, fruits and vegetables to provide the majority of your daily carbohydrate needs. Higher sugar foods such as candy, beverages and desserts can still be part of your overall carbohydrate intake, but they are not as nutritionally dense as other choices. If you are concerned about portion sizes, do use the information on the Nutrition Facts panel to discover what the serving size of your favorite food really is!

** If you are a vegetarian, you will still need to get your protein needs met. If meat, poultry or fish are not part of your diet, you will have to add extra dairy foods as well as beans, nuts and soy to meet your needs. Vegetables and grains can also provide protein, but in relatively small amounts. Do be aware that protein portions of plant-based foods are larger than animal products, so be sure to include an appropriate amount of these foods at every meal. If you do not use dairy foods, be sure to select soy products that have added calcium to keep your bones healthy.

*** Fat is an essential nutrient and should be part of your daily diet. Fat also promotes satiety to keep you from being overly hungry between meals, and it makes foods taste good too. Certain fats also may have health-promoting benefits. They include olive, canola, safflower, and peanut oil, nuts, and nut butters. Do try to include one or more of these foods daily. On the other hand, saturated fat foods such as bacon, cream cheese and sour cream are not as good for your health and should be used sparingly. There is NO nutritional advantage to fat-free fats such as spreads and salad dressings, other than the fact that they may save you a few calories. Do your taste buds a favor and use light or regular salad dressings or spreads, but be portion-savvy.

One of the other very important times for fueling is after exercise. What you eat, and when you eat after exercise can speed up or slow down recovery. For athletes who may have several events in one day or two-a-day practices or workouts, waiting too long to refuel is a recipe for disaster by the time the next practice rolls around. The optimal time to refuel is within 15 minutes after exercise. This doesn't mean that you have to sit down to a meal, but before you leave the gym, playing field, or hit the shower, you are going to want to put something into your body.

The goal is to be prepared. When you pack your exercise gear, throw in a portable snack that you can eat when your workout is over. If you drive to a practice or event or are going to pick up exercising kids, keep some snacks in the car. Snack size packages of goldfish crackers, animal crackers, pretzels, granola or cereal bars are excellent choices and best of all, they won't spoil even in a hot car or gym bag!

Good choices for after exercise would include about 50 grams of carbohydrate. Table 18.5 lists some good post exercise choices. Make sure that you pack something in your sports bag that you can easily grab after exercise, and make this a habit after every workout. The longer you wait to refuel, the longer it takes your body to recover.

Although you might not think of fluid as a fuel for exercise, drinking enough is essential for optimal exercise performance. If you don't drink enough fluid, you will experience the following:

- Decreased ability to concentrate
- Decreased strength
- Decreased speed
- Decreased endurance
- Decreased metabolic rate (the body does not burn calories at an efficient rate)
- Increased risk of injury

If you're thirsty, you are already dehydrated. The goal is to drink enough throughout the day. Don't wait until nighttime to drink. Not only will you find it difficult to drink all the fluid your body needs, but you'll be up all night long!

I also recommend that you weigh in and out before and after exercise. This is not to torture you, but to help you determine how

TABLE 18.5: 50 Gram Carbohydrate Food Choices for Use Post Exercise

FOOD	AMOUNT	CARBOHYDRATE (grams)
Cocoa Puffs	2 cups	54
Swedish Fish	½ cup	50
4 oz bagel with with 1tbsp jelly	½	52
Cereal bar	2	52
Yogurt	8 oz.	41
Pretzels	1 cup	44
Raisins	½ cup	60
Sports drink	32 oz.	60

much fluid you are losing during activity. Believe me, this is not fat loss, and whatever fluid you lose, you need to replace! You don't have to do this before every practice or event, but it is a good idea to do this for a few days, every couple of months, and especially when the weather gets hot and humid, and your fluid losses may increase.

The recommendations for fluid intake are as follows:

For an active female, you need to drink a minimum of your weight (in pounds) x 0.67 for the number of ounces of fluid your body requires daily. It is good idea to keep track of your current fluid intake as a baseline. Then you will know how close you are to meeting your needs, or how much work you have to do to get there. One of the most common mistakes made is to increase fluid too much and too quickly. Not only is this uncomfortable, but you will not be able to sustain this level of fluid consumption for any long period of time.

Let's say that you weigh 120 pounds. Your fluid needs are 80 (.67 x 120) ounces of fluid a day. This is the equivalent of four 20 ounce water bottles over the course of the day. After keeping a record for a few days, you determine that you are currently drinking 40 ounces of fluid. A good strategy would be the following:

WEEK 1: 40 ounces a day
WEEK 2: 48 ounces a day
WEEK 3: 56 ounces a day

WEEK 4: 64 ounces a day
WEEK 5: 72 ounces a day
WEEK 6: 80 ounces a day

Not only will this be more comfortable for you, but this type of drinking strategy will prevent you from spending all day in the bathroom instead of doing your sport!

Keep in mind that these are fluid requirements for an active woman at rest. You also need to keep yourself hydrated for activity. Fluid needs for exercise as follows:

16 ounces or 2 cups of fluid 2 hours before exercise
8 ounces of fluid 5-10 minutes before exercise*
4-8 ounces of fluid every 15-20 minutes during exercise**

** If you are going to be exercising for long periods of time*

*** 3-4 ounces for younger individuals*

Drink 24 ounces of fluid for every pound lost during exercise within 2 hours after exercise is done

In terms of fluid choices, women are much better about drinking water than men, but water alone may not be enough. Active women are more susceptible to lower blood sodium levels, which can detract from performance. You may want to consider using a sports drink before, during and after exercise to provide the body not only fluid, but fuel, as well as the electrolytes sodium and potassium. This may be especially important during prolonged exercise.

Milk, juice, and even coffee and tea provide fluid to the body, and all fruits and vegetables are 90-95 percent water. Soup, gelatin, and fruit ices are also fluid sources. Carbonated beverages are not the best choices simply because they can make you feel full before your body's fluid requirements are satisfied. I am not suggesting that you eliminate soda all together, but it is probably wise to choose other beverages especially before exercise.

Young girls, teens and older women need to pay extra attention to fluid needs, as the body's thirst mechanism may not adequately indicate when your body needs to drink. A good rule of thumb is to drink often, and drink plenty, and push yourself to consume 1-2 extra good sized gulps every time you have something to drink. Never shortchange your body when it comes to fluid needs. Not only will your fitness suffer, but your health will too.

Special Nutrient Requirements for Females

In addition to food and fluid choices, active females of all ages need to pay extra attention to meeting calcium and iron requirements. Calcium is critical for optimal bone health, but unfortunately, 50 percent of adolescent and adult females do not meet the daily calcium needs. Since the body cannot make calcium, food choices and/or supplementation is the only way to guarantee adequate intake.

Calcium needs based upon the Daily Reference Intakes are listed in Table 18.6. The tolerable upper limit of calcium for adults is 2500 milligrams per day, so more is of no additional benefit.

Dairy products are the most concentrated source of calcium, but they are not the only source. Foods that contain calcium provide calories, protein, carbohydrate, riboflavin (a B vitamin), vitamin D, potassium, phosphorus, and magnesium, in contrast to supplements, which only provide minerals. Calcium supplementation can be used to ensure that optimal daily needs are met, but should not be the sole source of calcium unless you are unable to meet your needs through diet. Table 18.7 lists the calcium content of various foods.

If you are finding it hard to meet daily calcium needs through foods alone, you may want to consider a calcium supplement to help you to meet your requirements. There are several products on the marketplace. Here are some guidelines for getting the most out of your product.

- Consider a calcium, vitamin D and vitamin K mixture.
- Do not take more than 500 milligrams of calcium at one time.
- Take your supplement with food.
- Look for the USP symbol on your supplement as a sign of better absorption.
- Stay away from products derived from bone meal, dolomite or oyster shells, which can contain lead.

In addition to meeting calcium needs, it is also important for active females to consume adequate iron. Menstruating females are at a higher risk of iron deficiency than men or non-menstruating women due to menstrual blood loss. Table 18-5 lists the iron requirements. The tolerable upper limit is 45 milligrams per day.

Iron is available to the body from animal sources, heme iron,

TABLE 18.6: Calcium Requirements by Age

AGE GROUP	*DRI Calcium (mg)*
Children	
4-8	800
18-18	1300
Women	
19-49	1000
Pregnant/Lactating	
< 18	1300
19-50	1000
Women over age 50	1200
Postmenopausal women not on estrogen	1500

plant sources and non heme iron. Table 18-9 lists the iron content of various foods.

Note that even if you choose not to include meat in your diet, there are many excellent plant-based iron sources. In order to maximize absorption of plant base iron foods, do try to do the following:

- Consume vitamin C containing foods such as orange juice or tomato products.
- Consider cooking tomato sauce in a cast iron skillet to boost iron intake.
- Choose breads, cereals and pastas with the words "iron-enriched" or "fortified" on the label.
- Do not drink coffee or tea with meals, which can interfere with iron absorption. Drink these beverages one hour before or after meals.

WEIGHT MANAGEMENT

I have many clients who are extremely physically fit, yet are totally done in by a number they see on the scale. An obsession with a particular weight or body fat percentage can prevent you from performing optimally. Keep in mind that no one can see what you weigh, but toned muscles, confidence and a YES I CAN attitude can be very apparent to yourself and to others.

TABLE 18.7: Calcium Sources

FOOD	*SERVING SIZE*	*CALCIUM(mg)*
Salmon (canned w/bones)	3 oz. can	503
Non-fat yogurt	8 oz. container	452
Low-fat yogurt	8 oz. container	415
Calcium-fortified frozen yogurt	1 cup	415
Calcium–fortified cottage cheese	1 cup	400
Non fat dry milk powder	¼ cup	377
Sardines (canned w/bones)	3 oz. can	372
Calcium fortified rice*	½ cup cooked	350
Calcium fortified orange juice*	8 oz. glass	350
Milk	8 oz. glass	300
Power Bar	2.3 oz.	300
Blackstrap molasses	2 tbsp.	274
Clif Luna Bar	1.7 oz.	260
Dried figs	5	258
PR Bar	1.76 oz.	250
Rice milk, fortified*	1 cup	240
Soy nuts*	½ cup	232
Tofu (with calcium salts)*	3 oz.	225
Carnation Instant Breakfast	1 packet	200
Calcium fortified soy milk*	1 cup	200-500
Calcium fortified cereals	1 oz.	200-250
Soy cheese, fortified*	1 oz.	200-300
Cheese	1 oz.	160-300
Corn meal, enriched, dry*	1/3 cup	140
Parmesan cheese, grated	2 tbsp.	138
Corn bread	2 oz piece	133
Tahini (sesame see paste)*	2 tbsp.	128
Turnip greens, cooked*	½ cup	99
Almonds*	¼ cup	94
Kale, cooked*	½ cup	90
Soybeans, cooked	½ cup	86
Vegetarian baked beans*	½ cup	64
Collard greens, cooked*	½ cup	64
Hummus*	½ cup	62
Orange*	1 medium	56
Corn tortilla	1, 6-inch diameter	53

* Plant sources of calcium

TABLE 18.8: Daily Iron Requirements

AGE	*IRON (mg)*
Premenopausal women	18
Pregnant women	27
Breast feeding/non-menstruating	9
Adolescent/breast feeding	10
Post-menopausal	8

If you are interested in losing body fat, remember that these changes take place over time. It is a good idea to have your body fat tested first so that you can make realistic changes to your eating. A good body fat level is one that is associated with consistent good performance and promotes good health. The lowest body fat percentage does not always result in the best athlete. Drastic alterations in eating are very stressful to the body and are too difficult to be maintained over an extended period of time. If you cut your calories too quickly or by too much, you will be tired, unable to think well, and your workouts will suffer too. Those who are most successful are willing to gradually modify food choices and eating behavior to have enough energy available to meet fitness and eating goals. Here are some tips to help you achieve your goals.

- Try to cut no more than 250-300 calories from your current daily caloric intake.
- Make sure you eat smaller more frequent meals, you will be less hungry.
- Watch some of the extras, such as salad dressings or sauces.
- Look at the Nutrition Facts panel for the portion size information.
- Include foods that take longer to eat — fruit, soups, salads.
- Boost up on your fiber intake through food, not supplements.
- Get calories from foods instead of liquids.
- Eat in response to hunger.
- Stop when you have had enough.
- Include foods that you like.
- Make eating purposeful, see what you eat.

TABLE 18.10: Iron Content of Foods

FOOD	*SERVING SIZE*	*IRON (mg)*
Heme iron		
Beef	3 oz.	2.5-3.5
Chicken, breast	3 oz.	1
Chicken, dark meat	3 oz.	1
Chicken livers	3 oz.	7
Fish	3 oz.	1
Pork	3 oz.	1
Non-heme iron		
Bread	1 slice	1
Beans, dried	½ cup cooked	1.5-2.5
Cereals, fortified	1 oz.	5-9
Cereals 100% fortified	1 oz.	10-15
Cream of Wheat	¾ cup cooked	8
Oatmeal	1 cup cooked	1.7
Spinach	½ cup cooked	3
Blackstrap molasses	1 tbsp.	3.5
Flour tortilla	10-inch	2.5
Sunflower seeds	1 oz.	2.2
Hummus	½ cup	2
Pasta	1 cup cooked	1.4
Prunes	5 large	1.7
Raisins	1 oz.	1
Brown rice	1 cup cooked	0.8

✳ Set realistic, do-able goals that you aim to achieve over a reasonable period of time.

✳ Consider working with a registered dietitian who can tailor a plan to meet your needs.

There are some active females who need to put on weight, and it can be as frustrating as those who are trying to shed pounds. To add mass you must increase your daily caloric intake above the current level. A good rule of thumb is to try to add 500 additional calories every day. Here are some tips to help with weight gain.

✳ Every food or beverage must have calories.

- ✳ Substitute higher calorie foods for lower calorie ones, ie. granola instead of wheat flakes, or a bagel instead of bread.
- ✳ Add ¼ more at every meal and snack.
- ✳ Eat frequently throughout the day.
- ✳ Make it a point to add calories every day of the week.
- ✳ If you increase your activity, you will need to increase your calorie intake as well.

The Bottom Line

Being in good body balance requires a combination of physical, mental and nutritional well-being. You owe it to yourself to give your body what it needs to be an active female. Do try to keep the following points in mind.

- ✳ Eating should be a pleasant, enjoyable experience.
- ✳ Make mealtimes relaxing.
- ✳ Space food out over the course of the day
- ✳ Eat a mix of foods at every meal and snack.
- ✳ Drink throughout the day.
- ✳ Remember, there are no bad foods, only bad attitudes.
- ✳ If your goal is to make changes to diet, make them gradually, one at a time.

Eat well to play well and live well.

RESOURCES

The American Dietetic Association
1-800 366-1655
www.eatright.org

SCAN -The Sports, Cardiovascular and Wellness Nutritionist Practice group of the American Dietetic Association
(719) 395-9271

www.NutriFit.org
Healthy Weight Network
1-701-567-2646
www.healthyweight.net

Gatorade Sports Science Institute
www.gssiweb.com

Section IV
Becoming Fit: Special Conditions

Fitness knows no boundaries.
– Joe Luxbacher

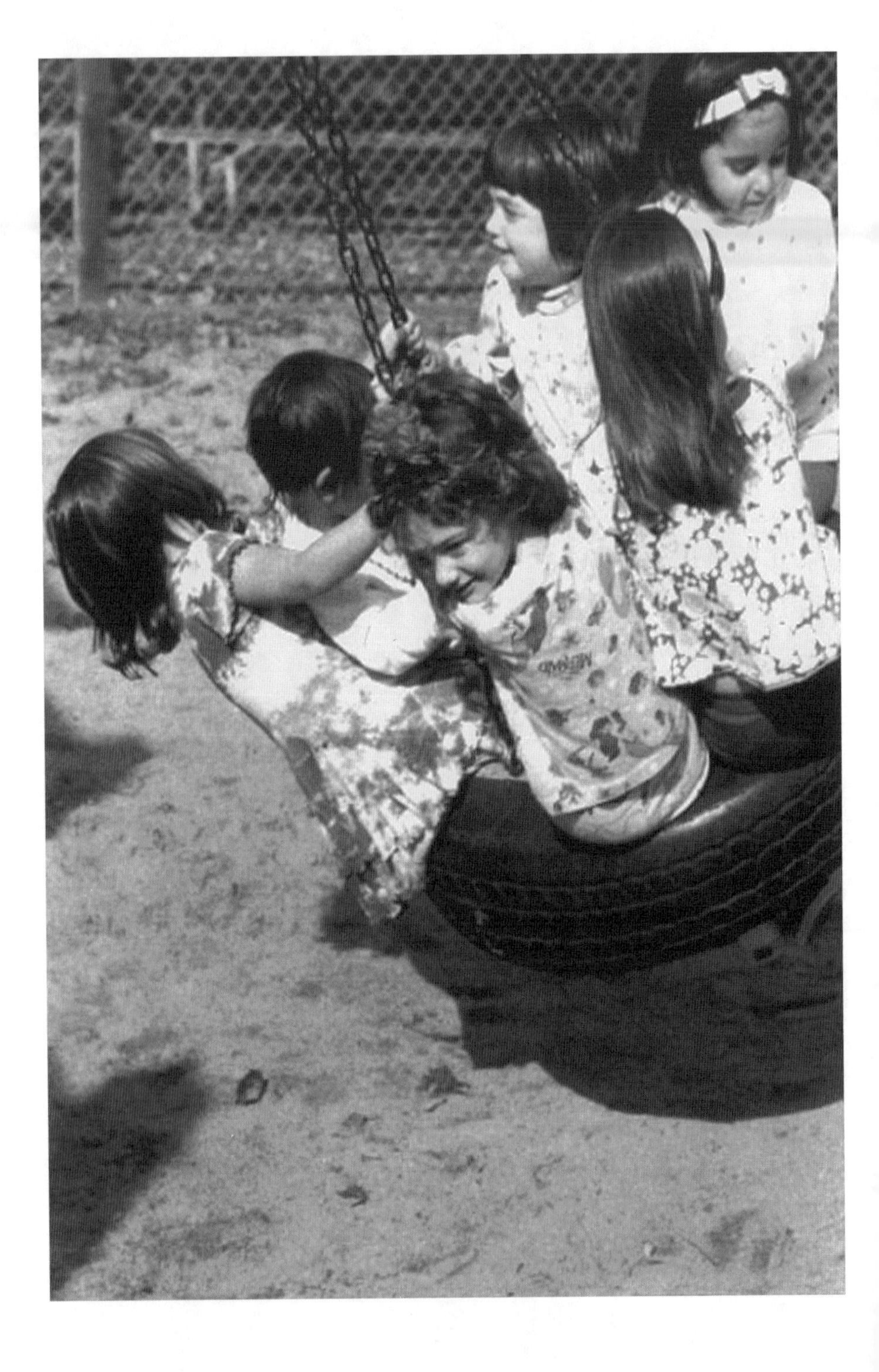

Kids and Fitness 19

Children today are heavier and less fit than just a decade ago. One in four are overweight. The majority do not measure up to minimal standards for strength and endurance. Childhood obesity is increasing in leaps and bounds. I could go on. The primary forces driving these trends are obvious. Our kids are eating too much and exercising too little. Children today consume approximately 200 calories more per day than they did 10 years ago. Even if activity levels were the same now as then, and they are not, that still translates into a heck of a lot of extra body fat. The problem is magnified by the fact that kids today are even less active! Only one in three participate in daily exercise of any kind. The typical toddler spends three hours or more each day sitting in front of the TV. Grade-school children spend nearly as much time watching television and playing video games as they do in school. To make matters worse, studies show that physical activity in children declines steadily with age. Exercise for many teenagers consists solely of manipulating electronically-held video games. While this may do wonders for finger dexterity, it doesn't do much for their heart, muscles and circulatory system.

The growing trend towards pre-adolescent couch potatoes has long-reaching ramifications. Although many parents view "baby fat" as merely a passing phase in their child's life, for many kids it actually signals the beginning of a lifelong struggle with obesity. It's a fact that overweight children are more likely to become overweight adults.

Habits Learned Early Can Shape a Life (and a Body!)

Children aren't born with an inherent sweet tooth or propensity for inactivity. Eating and exercise habits are *learned behaviors*. A child's perception of exercise and physical activity in general, is influenced by a variety of sources. Although teachers, peers, television, and the print media all play a role, parents ultimately shoulder the bulk of responsibility. Modeling is a powerful learning tool so it is imperative that mom and dad set a good example. Studies

TABLE 19.1: Overweight Children and Adolescents as a Percent of the U.S. Population

BOYS	*1963-65*	*1971-74*	*1976-80*	*1988-94*
6-8 yrs	5.1	6.3	8.1	15.4
9-11 yrs	4.8	6.7	8.1	14
12-14 yrs	5.2	5.4	5.4	11.5
15-17 Yrs	4.8	5.2	5.1	13.1

GIRLS	*1963-65*	*1971-74*	*1976-80*	*1988-94*
6-8 yrs	5.1	4.1	7.1	14.6
9-11 yrs	5.2	4.7	7.1	10.8
12-14 yrs	5.0	8.6	7.8	13.9
15-17 Yrs	4.9	6.0	4.5	7.5

Source: Centers for Disease Control and Prevention

show that parents who are physically active have a six times greater chance of developing lifelong exercise habits in their children. Lecturing a child to eat responsibly and exercise regularly won't carry much weight if she sees firsthand that her parents place little value on physical activity and healthy eating habits. If you have kids, like I do, you can attest to the fact that children are poor listeners but great imitators.

Children and Exercise: What Kind and How Much?

Children are not miniature adults. Their bodies will not respond to exercise in the same ways as ours, and they cannot safely handle the same relative workload. Their circulatory system and muscles are not fully developed and bones are still being formed. Any form of exercise that puts undue stress on bones, joints, muscles and the cardiorespiratory system is not appropriate. In simple terms, kids shouldn't run too hard, jump too high or lift too much weight. The overriding goal of a children's fitness program should be the development of positive exercise habits that will carry into adulthood. The emphasis should be on long-term benefits as opposed to short-term performance gains.

Cardiovascular Fitness. There is some question as to how much children will benefit from formal aerobic training. The few studies that are available suggest that cardiovascular fitness in young children does not improve as much as would be expected. Significant gains appear to occur only after children have reached puberty. With that in mind, everyday activities such as running after a ball, riding a bike, climbing a jungle-gym, hiking in the woods and participating in dance class are preferred over structured fitness training. Kids who are physically active on a daily basis don't require a formal exercise program to stay healthy and in-shape

Weight Training. The issue of whether strength training is appropriate for prepubescent children remains a hot topic of discussion among parents, coaches and sport scientists. In the not-so-distant past girls, even more so than boys, were discouraged from lifting weights for fear that improper technique would damage the growth center of developing bones. Current research has alleviated those concerns. The American Academy of Pediatrics, the American College of Sports Medicine, and the National Strength and Conditioning Association all support appropriately designed and supervised strength training programs for children.

Children will gain strength faster by lifting a light- to moderate amount of resistance for many repetitions as opposed to working with heavier weights. This approach differs from that generally adopted by adults, who build muscle most effectively by lifting heavy weights for fewer repetitions. If hand-held free weights

Weight Training Guidelines for Children

Prepubescent children participating in a weight training program should adhere to the following guidelines set forth by the American College of Sports Medicine (ACSM).

- Adequate supervision at all times by knowledgeable individuals.
- Perform all exercises through a full range of motion.
- No maximum lifts attempted.
- Two to three training sessions per week are recommended. Twenty to thirty minutes per session.
- Select a weight that the child can perform 6 to 15 repetitions per set.
- Perform one to three sets per exercise.
- The resistance can be increased in one- to three- pound increments after the child can perform 15 repetitions in correct form.

(dumbbells, barbells) aren't available, children can use their own body weight as the resistance to be pushed, pulled or lifted. A variety of modified push-ups, pull-ups, dips and abdominal exercises can provide the same basic strength benefits as free-weight training, and the likelihood of accidental injury is less.

What to Do When Your Child is Overweight

Given the choice no child wants to be overweight, but she or he won't solve the problem alone. Parents must take an active role in providing guidance, support and understanding. The following tips will help in that process.

1. ***Provide leadership***. In most cases kids will not make intelligent food choices. They want what tastes best to them, which usually means a high-fat high-sugar content treat. It is the parent's responsibility to provide healthy meals and nutritious snacks.
2. ***No forbidden foods***. Everyone craves "junk food" once in a while. View your child's diet in its entirety; treats are okay so long as the bulk of their diet is healthy
3. ***Encourage physical activity***. (See the following section on "motivating kids to be active.")
4. ***Turn off the television***. The American Academy of Pediatrics recommends limiting TV time to less than two hours per day.
5. ***Don't diet!*** Cutting back drastically on calories may result in a child not getting enough essential nutrients. The key to achieving normal body weight is to eat healthy and sensibly.
6. ***Limit high calorie drinks***. Juices and soda are two of the primary culprits. Kids are better off eating fruit than drinking fruit-flavored drinks and drinking soda is the equivalent of drinking a bottle of sugar water.
7. ***Avoid quick fixes***. Aim for permanent behavior changes that result in gradual weight loss of ½ pound per week.

Motivating Kids to Be Active

It doesn't take a rocket scientist to figure out that children are more likely to repeat an activity if they enjoy it. They will also be more likely to do it spontaneously, without adult coaxing or supervision. If we expect our kids to be active on a regular basis, it is essential that they equate exercise with fun. Improved health and fitness should be viewed as an added benefit, not necessarily the ultimate goal. While participation in school-sponsored programs such as T-ball, soccer and basketball are viable ways of getting children to move about, they are by no means the only ways. Children must be motivated to exercise on their own. The following exercise turn-ons can help to achieve that aim:

- Choose activities that have a high recreational component.
- Provide an opportunity for each child to achieve some degree of success. No one likes to be embarrassed or view themselves as a failure.
- Make exercise a family affair. Hiking, biking, swimming and cross-country skiing are activities that the entire family can do together
- Make physical activity a social affair. Organize fitness-related parties, such as a group ice skating event or camping trip.
- Attend a sport camp. Kids will not only benefit from learning sport-specific skills that can lead to future sport participation, but they may also develop friendships that can have a positive influence on their lives.

Our Responsibility as Parents

Although we can't change genes, we can change habits. Our children will benefit from breaking a sweat in the same ways as you or I. An improved level of fitness will positively influence other areas of a child's life as well, such as enhanced self-esteem and self-confidence. The youth of America are not destined to be overweight, under fit and unhealthy. When we provide our kids with an appreciation and love of physical activity we have truly given them a priceless gift, one that will enhance the quality of their life for years to come.

Exercise and Pregnancy 20

Women who exercise may eventually have to make an important decision — whether or not to continue their workouts during pregnancy. While there is no guarantee that regular exercise will improve the outcome of a pregnancy, there are several potential benefits. By remaining active you will maintain muscle strength and endurance, which should make it easier (if that is possible!) to carry around the extra weight. Strong muscles help to promote good posture which can alleviate discomforts such as lower back pain, fatigue, bloating and swelling. Exercise can provide a psychological boost to counteract feelings of stress, anxiety and depression. Last but certainly not least, regular exercise can promote a readiness for labor. The physically fit woman is likely to experience a faster recovery from labor and will usually find it easier to get back into game shape after the baby arrives.

Too much of a good thing may not be good however. There are several hypothetical concerns associated with *heavy exercise* during pregnancy. These include 1) reduced blood flow to the uterus which can result in insufficient oxygen supplied to the fetus; a condition referred to as *fetal hypoxia;* 2) elevated fetal temperature associated with the mother's increased body temperature in response to prolonged aerobic exercise, a condition referred to as *fetal hyperthermia;* 3) reduced carbohydrate (glucose) availability to the fetus because the mother's body uses available carbohydrates to fuel exercise; 4) reduced birth weight; and 5) the possibility of miscarriage or premature labor. It is unclear whether any of these concerns are legitimate. You can alleviate any reservations you may have by using caution and common sense.

Playing It Safe

The American College of Obstetricians and Gynecologists (ACOG) differentiate between women who exercise and become pregnant, and those who begin to exercise during pregnancy. ACOG recommends that women who already exercise on a regular basis continue to do so during pregnancy, although they should gradually decrease the duration and intensity of their workouts as the pregnancy advances. Women who were not exercising prior to pregnancy should get permission from their physician before starting a program. Once cleared, they can begin with low-intensity low-impact aerobics such as walking or stationary cycling.

- *Maternal Heart Rate*. The average woman gains 20 to 35 pounds during her pregnancy. Carrying around the extra weight will require you to work harder, even when exercising at a slower pace, so you do not want to overdo it. It's a good idea to monitor your heart rate at times of peak activity. The ACOG recommends that the maternal heart rate not exceed 140 beats per minute when exercising. *(Note: See Chapter 11 Aerobic Fitness to learn how to monitor heart rate.)*
- ***Type of Exercise.*** Pregnancy causes a variety of changes in a woman's body, internally as well as externally. Your center of gravity will gradually shift as the pregnancy progresses. Hormonal changes cause connective tissues to soften and may produce joint instability. Certain types of exercise become inappropriate, either because they are too intense or because they involve movements that are uncomfortable to the mother or harmful to the fetus. Avoid high impact, bouncy-type movements, as well as full sit-ups and straight-leg toe touches. As a general rule, no exercise should be performed in the supine (back on the floor) position after the fourth month.
- ***Fetal Hyperthermia.*** It has been proposed, although not proven, that an elevated body temperature during early pregnancy can result in birth defects. As a precautionary measure pregnant women should avoid overheating, usually defined as a body temperature in excess of 100 degrees Fahrenheit. Vigorous aerobic exercise, particularly in hot and humid environments, should be avoided. Because dehydration will also raise core body temperature, an expectant mother should drink ample amounts of fluid before and after exercising.

Exercise Guidelines During Pregnancy

The ACOG offers the following guidelines for the development of a safe exercise program during pregnancy and postpartum periods.

- Obtain medical clearance prior to beginning any exercise program. Your doctor can assist in choosing the most appropriate exercises and activities.
- Regular exercise (at least three days per week) is preferable to intermittent activity. Competitive sports are not recommended.
- Non-weight bearing exercise such as cycling and swimming is preferable to weight-bearing exercise such as jogging and skipping rope.
- Avoid exercise that requires jumping, bouncing or rapid changes of direction. Deep flexion and extension of the joints is discouraged.
- Perform a warm-up prior to exercise. You can do this by walking slowly or pedaling the stationary bike at a very low resistance.
- Avoid strenuous exercise during the first trimester.
- Avoid prolonged vigorous exercise in warm, humid environments.
- Drink an ample amount of fluids before and after exercise to ensure adequate hydration.
- Do not exercise when fatigued, particularly during late pregnancy.
- If unusual symptoms appear, such as pain, dizziness, rapid heart beat at rest, vaginal bleeding, or shortness of breath, stop exercising at once and contact your physician.

In summary, the benefits of exercise during pregnancy greatly outweigh the risks when caution and common sense are applied. In all cases a woman should coordinate her program with an obstetrician who can provide guidance in choosing the most appropriate types of activities. For additional information see: *Exercise and Fitness: A Guide for Women (1992). The American College of Obstetricians and Gynecologists.*

You're Never Too Old! 21

It is not surprising that a growing number of older adults are adopting a physically active lifestyle. The evidence shows clearly that exercise isn't just a kid thing. Even if you are in your 70s or 80s and haven't been active in years, embarking on a program of moderately-intense physical activity will improve your health and lengthen your life. While the fittest people tend to live the longest, the biggest jump in life expectancy occurs with those who go from doing nothing to doing something.

Regular exercise provides the key that can unlock your personal fountain of youth. It can reverse, or at the very least slow, many of the physical and mental changes we associate with aging. The Centers for Disease Control and Prevention recommend that adults of all ages accumulate a minimum of 30 minutes or more of moderate-intensity activity on most days of the week. Walking, cycling and swimming definitely fit the bill, as do more functional activities such as raking leaves, gardening and mowing the lawn. The bottom line is this. Regardless of age, it is in your best interests to get your body moving on a regular basis. There is nothing else you can do that will have as positive an effect on the quality of your life.

By age 70 without regular exercise ...

- Our lungs can lose up to one-half of their breathing capacity
- Pumping efficiency of the heart can decrease by as much as one-third.
- Bones lose density and become more brittle; the likelihood of fractures increase.
- The average woman loses 30 percent or more of her muscle mass.
- Normal household chores like carrying out the garbage become more difficult.
- Metabolism slows. We gain fat and our immune system weakens.

Aerobic Exercise and Older Adults

The wide range of health and fitness levels present in older adults makes it difficult to prescribe a program appropriate for everyone.The following recommendations are adapted from American College of Sports Medicine guidelines and can be used to establish the type, intensity, duration, and frequency of aerobic workouts.

Type of Exercise

- Chose activities that do not create significant orthopedic stress.
- Choose activities that are convenient and enjoyable.
- Excellent choices include walking, stationary biking, machine-based stair climbing, swimming, and water-based exercise.

Intensity of Exercise

- Sufficient to stress the cardiovascular, pulmonary, and musculoskeletal systems without overtaxing them.
- Because there is high variability for maximal heart rates in persons over 65 years of age, it is recommended that a measured maximal heart rate be used rather than an age-predicted maximal heart rate.
- The Karvonen heart rate reserve method *(See Chapter 15)* is

TABLE 21.1: Age Group Participation in Fitness Activities

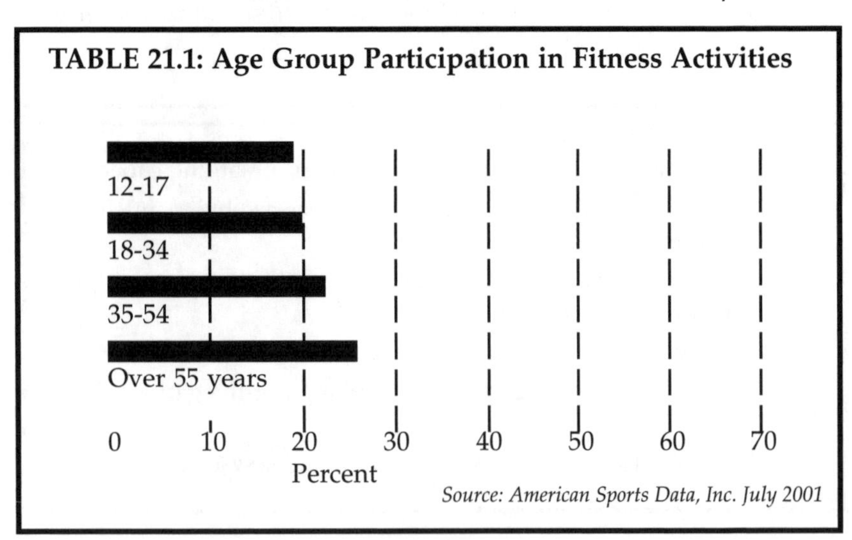

Source: American Sports Data, Inc. July 2001

recommended for establishing a training heart rate in older adults, as opposed to a straight percentage of heart rate.

* Recommended exercise intensity for older adults is 50 to 70% of heart rate reserve.
* A conservative approach is recommended.

Duration of Exercise

* Some older adults will have difficulty sustaining aerobic exercise for 20 minutes or more. If that is the case you can perform exercise in multiple 10-minute bouts throughout the day.
* Initially increase exercise duration rather than intensity.

Frequency of Exercise

* Alternate between days that involve weight bearing and non-weight bearing exercise.

Strength Training and Older Adults

The typical woman will lose about 1 percent of her muscle mass for each year after the age of 30. Muscles gradually become weaker and less defined. Metabolism slows. Bones become weaker and more brittle. Loss of balance occurs more frequently which increases the likelihood of falls and broken bones. In short, the quality of life declines. For these reasons the importance of minimizing strength loss as we get older cannot be overstated. Weight training can do this and as a consequence may actually be more important than aerobic exercise for older adults.

The following strength-training guidelines apply to the majority of older women. Special conditions, such as a history of heart disease or high blood pressure, should be evaluated on an individual basis through consultation with a physician.

Intensity

* Perform one set of 8 to10 exercises that target all of the major muscle groups.
* Perform 8 to 12 repetitions per set.

Frequency

* At least twice per week, with 48 hours or more between workouts.

Duration

- ✻ A total body program of 20 to 30 minutes should be sufficient.

How Hard Should You Exercise?

What constitutes a moderately-intense level of physical activity? It depends on your level of fitness. A relatively light workload for the fit individual may be extremely rigorous for the unfit person. You can determine whether you are exercising in your aerobic training zone (50 to 70 percent of heart rate reserve) by monitoring heart rate (*See Chapter 15*), or simply through perceptions of how you feel during the exercise. You can do this using the *Borg Ratings of Perceived Exertion Scale (Table 21.2).*

The numbers on the left column of the Borg Scale provide an estimate of perceived exertion, or how hard you feel you are work-

TABLE 21.2: The Borg Category Rating Scale

Rating	Description	Training
Least Effort		
6		
7	Very very light	
8		
9	Very light	
10		
11	Fairly light	Aerobic Training (11–13)
12		
13	Somewhat hard	
14		
15	Hard	
16		
17	Very hard	Strength Training (17–19)
18		
19	Very, very hard	
20		
Maximum Effort		

ing. When performing aerobic exercise older adults should gradually work up to a perceived exertion level of between 11 and 13. For some that may equate with a brisk walk; for others it may require jogging at a 9-minute per mile pace. In all cases the exercise should not make you breathe so hard that you can't talk. Developing your muscles will require a slightly higher level of exercise intensity. When strength training, gradually work up to a perceived exertion range of 15 to 17 (hard to very hard). *Because individuals may respond differently to the same volume of exercise, the Borg Scale is not as accurate as heart monitoring when it comes to estimating exercise intensity.*

Flexibility and Older Adults

We become less flexible as we get older due to reduced activity levels and a reduction in the elasticity of our muscles and connective tissues. To an extent stretching exercises will counteract normal declines in flexibility. Perform all stretches in a smooth and controlled manner, and never stretch a muscle beyond its pain-free range of motion. Pain is a warning signal that you are doing too much! Older adults should consider the following guidelines** when stretching.

Intensity

- Slowly extend the muscle(s) to a full stretch position until experiencing a feeling tightness or mild discomfort.
- Hold each stretch for 15 to 30 seconds.
- Cover every major joint (hip, back, shoulder, knee, upper trunk and neck) in the body.
- Perform three to five repetitions of each stretch.

Frequency

- Stretch at least three times per week (preferably daily).

Duration

- The stretching portion of a workout session should last 10 to 20 minutes.
- Devoting an entire workout to flexibility may be appropriate for totally sedentary, unfit older adults who are just beginning an exercise program.

Always warm-up with several minutes of light aerobic exercise prior to stretching. Activities such as walking or cycling will

increase blood circulation and raise core body temperature.
**Adapted from ACSM Guidelines for Exercise Testing and Prescription

Exercise and the Environment 22

The environmental factors of heat, cold and air pollution can impact the quality and, in some cases, safety of your workouts. The following material discusses potential dangers of exercising in extreme conditions and provides common sense guidelines that will keep you safe, healthy and physically active.

Exercising in the Heat

The combined effect of four factors — *air temperature, humidity, wind velocity, and thermal radiation* — determine the amount of heat stress imposed on the body during exercise. For example, exercising on a sunny 80-degree day with no wind produces significantly greater thermal stress than exercising in the same temperature with a 15 mile-per-hour wind and heavy cloud cover. Likewise, you are more likely to overheat in 90-degree temperature at 95 percent humidity than at significantly lower humidity. High humidity impairs the body's natural cooling mechanism (sweating).

Heat-Related Problems

Heat cramps generally take the form of spasms in the muscles performing the bulk of the exercise. For example, it is not uncommon for a female soccer player to experience cramping in her calf or hamstring muscles during the later stages of a match played on a hot, humid day. Cramps result from dehydration and mineral losses incurred during heavy sweating, although other factors may also play a role.

Heat exhaustion occurs when the body's cooling systems fail to adequately dissipate heat. During heavy exercise a competition arises between the skin and muscles performing the work for a limited blood supply. Your muscles need oxygen carried by the blood to sustain the activity, while your skin uses blood to facilitate heat loss and keep your body cool. Heat exhaustion occurs when the cardiovascular system does not distribute an adequate supply of blood to the skin for heat dissipation, or when total blood volume decreases significantly due to fluid loss. Anyone can experi-

Figure 22.1: Heat Index Chart

Relative humidity (%)

temp	30	35	40	45	50	55	60	65	70	75	80	85	90	95	100
115	136	144	151												
110	123	138	137	141	158										
105	113	118	123	129	130	136	140								
100	104	107	110	115	120	126	135	144	148						
95	96	98	101	104	107	110	114	119	124	136	139				
90	90	91	93	95	96	98	100	102	106	109	113	117	122		
85	84	85	86	87	88	89	90	91	93	95	97	99	102	105	108
80	78	79	79	80	81	81	82	83	85	86	86	87	88	88	91
75	73	73	74	74	75	75	76	76	77	77	78	78	79	79	80
70	67	67	68	68	69	69	70	70	70	70	71	71	71	71	72

Caution Extreme caution Danger Extreme Danger

130°F or higher: Heatstroke/sunstroke highly likely with continued exposure

105° to 130°F: Sunstroke, heat cramps or heat exhaustion likely, and heatstroke possible with prolonged exposure and/or physical activity.

90° to 105°F: Sunstroke, heat cramps or heat exhaustion possible with prolonged exposure and/or physical activity.

Source: National Oceanic and Atmospheric Administration

ence heat exhaustion, although unfit individuals are most susceptible. Symptoms can include dizziness, breathlessness, cold and clammy skin, hot and dry skin, vomiting, fainting and rapid pulse. Heat exhaustion is a more serious condition than heat cramps. If unchecked, it can lead to heat stroke.

Heat stroke is a potentially life-threatening condition caused by a total collapse of the body's heat dissipating mechanisms. Symptoms include hot and dry skin, rapid pulse, a body temperature in excess of 104 degrees, confusion and unconsciousness. Rapid cooling of the body is critical to survival. This is usually done by placing the person in a bath of cold water or by wrapping her in wet sheets. Immediate attention by trained medical personnel is critical to survival.

Taking Precautions

Prevention is always preferred to after-the-fact treatment. Consider the following when exercising in hot, humid environments:

- ✳ Exercise early in the morning or later in the evening.
- ✳ Drink ample amounts of fluids, even more than thirst indicates (See Sidebar).
- ✳ Wear as little clothing as possible to allow heat exchange with the environment.
- ✳ **Do not** wear a rubberized suit in an effort to promote sweating and fat loss.
- ✳ Be aware of early warning signals and take appropriate action.

Exercising in the Cold

Any condition that causes significant loss of body heat poses a legitimate threat to your health. To avoid such problems our body has several built-in safeguards designed to conserve heat and increase heat production when needed. We've all experienced the most common of these mechanisms. *Shivering* is the involuntary contraction and relaxation of skeletal muscles that occurs when the brain senses a decrease in either skin or blood temperature. Shivering can increase the body's resting rate of heat production to several times that of normal.

Sport Drinks vs. Water?

Inadequate hydration is a concern for women who exercise regularly in hot, humid conditions. In most situations water will do fine as a replacement drink, particularly during short-term exercise. Drinking water does not compensate for electrolyte loss, however, which becomes more likely during prolonged endurance exercise. In that instance a carbohydrate (sport) drink can offer advantages. For one, sport drinks taste good so you are more likely to consume a greater quantity of fluid. This is important because thirst is not an accurate indicator of fluid needs. The thirst mechanism almost always *underestimates* fluid needs. The extra carbohydrate contained in sport drinks will also help to maintain blood glucose levels, which will enable you to exercise for longer periods of time without becoming fatigued.

Note: Sport drinks contain calories and plain water does not. A couple of glasses of a high-carb drink will replace most if not all of the calories burned during your workout. If you are trying to cut calories, good old-fashioned H2O is your best choice.

Cold-Related Problems

Hypothermia results from a massive loss of body heat. Humans must maintain a core body temperature within fairly narrow limits. A shift of just a few degrees either side of normal (98.6 degrees F) can spell serious trouble. When body temperature falls below 94 degrees F the hypothalmus portion of the brain begins to lose its ability to regulate body temperature. Metabolic reactions slow and drowsiness, or even coma, can occur. This is the feeling that reportedly overcomes mountain climbers exposed to the elements in sub-arctic conditions.

Frostbite occurs when the body reduces blood flow to the skin in an attempt to prevent heat loss. If unchecked the skin tissue eventually dies from lack of oxygen and nutrients. Exposed skin will freeze when its temperature is lowered below 32 degrees Fahrenheit (0 degrees Celsius). Due to the warming effects of circulation and metabolic heat production, the windchill required to freeze exposed skin is approximately minus 20 degrees F. Frostbite injuries can be serious if not treated immediately.

Figure 22.2 Windchill Factor Chart

Actual thermometer reading (°F)

Est. wind speed km/h	50	40	30	20	10	0	-10	-20	-30	-40	-50	-60
	Equivalent temperature (°F)											
Calm	50	40	30	20	10	0	-10	-20	-30	-40	-50	-60
8	48	37	27	16	6	-5	-15	-26	-36	-47	-57	-68
16.1	40	28	16	4	-9	-24	-33	-46	-58	-70	-83	-95
24.1	36	22	9	-5	-18	-32	-45	-58	-72	-85	-99	-112
32.2	32	18	4	-10	-25	-39	-53	-67	-82	-96	-110	-124
40.2	30	16	0	-15	-29	-44	-59	-74	-88	-104	-118	-133
48.3	28	13	-2	-18	-33	-48	-63	-79	-94	-109	-125	-140
56.3	27	11	-4	-20	-35	-51	-67	-82	-98	-113	-129	-145
64.4	26	10	-6	-21	-37	-53	-69	-85	-100	-116	-132	-148

Wind speeds greater than 64.4 km/h have little additional affect.

Light grey: little danger for properly clothed person. Maximum danger of false sense of security.

White: increasing danger from freezing of exposed flesh.

Dark grey: great danger.

Breathing Frigid Air

It is common misconception that breathing cold air will cause damage to the lungs and respiratory tract. In reality, cold air that passes into the mouth is warmed by the time it reaches the back of your nasal passage. Although excessive breathing of cold air through the mouth may cause mild irritation, it poses no real threat of damage to your throat or lungs.

Watch Out for Windchill

Air temperature alone is not an accurate measure of coldness. Windy conditions coupled with frigid temperatures, a measure commonly referred to as *windchill,* increases the rate of heat loss. Factor in humidity and you have the potential for serious problems (See Figure 22.2). Several years ago I experienced this phenomenon first-hand while climbing Mt. Washington in White Mountains of New Hampshire. When a friend and I began our climb at approximately 10 a.m. it was 60 degrees Fahrenheit and the sun was shining. As we reached the tree line a few hours later the temperature had dropped into the low 40s and strong winds were whipping moist clouds horizontally across the slopes. At that point of the climb we were dripping wet. I can vividly remember that my hands were so cold I couldn't tie the laces of my boot. Fortunately we reached the summit and the warmth of an Appalachian mountain hut before ending up in serious trouble. It was a learning experience I'll never forget.

Air Pollution

The automotive and industrial pollution common to major urban areas poses a legitimate health threat. While the harmful effects of air pollution have the greatest impact on the very young, the very old, and people with respiratory problems, long-term exposure to airborne pollutants can cause adverse effects to healthy, physically active adults as well. Because activities such as running, biking and skating increase the volume of air taken into the lungs both during and shortly after the workout, women who exercise regularly in highly polluted environments are placing themselves at risk.

Many airborne pollutants are relatively harmless when considered by themselves but become much more dangerous when intermixed with others. Combinations of common pollutants such as soot, ozone, sulfur dioxide and nitrous oxides have been linked to heart and lung disease, irritation of respiratory passages, suppression of immune system, and even some forms of cancer.

I am not suggesting that women who live in major urban areas should give up on exercise. The air quality around many of our major cities has actually improved over the past half century. My hometown of Pittsburgh, Pennsylvania, is a prime example, where the air is much cleaner now that it was during the heyday of the industrial revolution. In addition, the human respiratory system displays a remarkable ability to cleanse itself. Unless the air is highly polluted, our body does a pretty good job of protecting us from harmful effects. My advice would be to use common sense when deciding where and when to exercise. Avoid areas where pollution levels are likely to be highest, such as a ball field or track located next to a major expressway. Call the local weather station to check the air pollution index. On days when the pollution count is extremely high consider exercising indoors.

Commit to be Fit 23

Chapter 23 marks the end of one journey and the beginning of another. At this point you are prepared to add a new chapter to your life. You recognize the many benefits of being physically fit. You understand that becoming fit is a lifelong process involving a number of interconnected components. You realize the importance of planning, setting goals and identifying targets. You have an appreciation for the immense power of habit, and understand how you can harness that power to shape your physical destiny. You are aware of the potential pitfalls that lie between you and your fitness goals and are prepared to overcome them. In short, you now possess the skill, knowledge and motivation necessary to achieve total fitness. The next step is up to you.

The all-important catchword for realizing the many benefits that exercise has to offer is consistency. It's not what you do once in a while that makes a significant difference, but rather what you do on a regular basis that produces lasting results. This rule applies to virtually every aspect of your life. You have arrived at a fork in the road leading to your future and must decide on which path to follow. You can choose the road that will ultimately lead to physical and mental well being (you may already be on that road!), or you can ignore what you've learned and follow the path traveled by the overweight and under fit. For your sake and the sake of your family, I urge you to follow the road less traveled, the path that leads to lifelong health and fitness. Keep in mind that nothing positive results from a failure to act. Your immediate goal is to take that all-important first step on the road to becoming totally fit. I'm absolutely sure that you will enjoy the journey.

Be Happy. Be Healthy. Be Fit.

The Ten Commandments of Working Out

The following common sense guidelines are provided by the American Council on Exercise to assist individuals who are just beginning an exercise program.

1. Thou shalt stretch sufficiently. Before and after working out, take a few minutes to stretch muscles to prevent injury and stiffness.
2. Thou shalt not lift too much weight. Gradual, progressive resistance increases strength and prevents injury.
3. Thou shalt warm up. Take a few minutes to adjust to vigorous activity before jumping right in.
4. Thou shalt cool down. Take a few minutes to lower activity level and heart rate before calling it a day.
5. Thou shalt not overdo it. Don't try to cram a week's worth of exercise into one weekend afternoon.
6. Thou shalt hydrate. Drink fluids or risk injury or sickness.
7. Thou shalt not lean heavily on the aerobic stepper. Leaning on the machine defeats the purpose of using it for exercise.
8. Thou shalt workout rigorously. Don't overdo it, but under doing it isn't going to achieve the results you desire.
9. Thou shalt not lift weights jerkily. When lifting weights, smooth motion is the key to an effective and safe workout.
10. Eateth not energy bars nor drinketh sport beverages if the workout is less than two hours. These high-calorie products are only for those who really push it.

Appendices

Appendix A

Health and Fitness Organizational Contacts

ORGANIZATION	PHONE
Aerobic and Fitness Association of America	800-225-2322
Administration on Aging	202-619-0724
Amateur Athletic Union	800-AAU-4USA
American Academy of Pediatrics	847-228-5005
American Alliance for Health, Physical Education, Recreation & Dance	703-476-3400
American College of Sports Medicine	317-637-9200
American Heart Association	202-822-9380
American Orthopaedic Society for Sports Medicine	847-292-4900
American Running and Fitness Association	800-776-2732
Centers for Disease Control and Prevention Nutrition and Physical Activity Division	888-232-4674
National Association of Sport and Physical Education	800-321-0789
National Mental Health Association	703-684-7722
National Osteoporosis Foundation	800-223-9994
National Strength and Conditioning Association	719-632-6722
United States Olympic Committee	719-632-5551
Women's Sports Foundation	516-542-4700

APPENDIX B

The following organizations offer information about exercise and exercise programs.

American Academy of Orthopedic Surgeons
P.O. Box 1998
Des Plaines, IL 60017
Phone: 1-800-824-BONES

American College of Sports Medicine
P.O. Box 1440
Indianapolis, IN 46206
Internet: http://www.acsm.org

American Diabetes Association
1660 Duke Street
Alexandria, VA 22314
Phone 703-549-1500
Internet: http://www.diabetes.org

American Heart Association
National Center
7272 Greenville Avenue
Dallas, TX 75231-4596
Phone 1-800-AHA-USA1
Internet: http://www.Americanheart.org

American Physical Therapy Association
111 North Fairfax Street
Alexandria, VA 22314-1488
Phone 1-800-999-2782
Internet: http://www.apta.org

Arthritis Foundation
P.O. Box 7669
Atlanta, GA 30357-0669
Phone 1-800-283-7800
Internet: http://www.arthritis.org

The Cooper Institute for Aerobics Research
12330 Preston Road
Dallas, TX 75243
Internet: http://www.cooperinst.org

50-Plus Fitness Association
P.O. Box D
Stanford, CA 94309
Phone 650-323-6160
Internet: http://www.50plus.org

National Association of Governor's Councils on
Physical Fitness and Sports
Pan American Plaza
201 South Capitol Avenue, Suite 560
Indianapolis, IN 46225
Phone 317-237-5630
Internet: http://www.fitnesslink.com/Govcouncil/

National Institute on Aging/National Institutes of Health
Bldg. 31 Room 5C27
31 Center Drive, MSC 2292
Bethesda, MD 20892-2292
Phone 1-80-222-2225
Internet: http://www.nih.gov/nia

National Osteoporosis Foundation
1150 17th Street N.W., Suite 500
Washington, DC 20036
Phone 202-223-2226
Internet: http://www.nof.org

The President's Council on Physical Fitness and Sports
DHHS/OS/OPHS
200 Independence Avenue, S.W.
HHH Bldg., Room 738H
Washington, DC 20201
Phone 202-690-9000
Internet: http://www.os.dhhs.gov

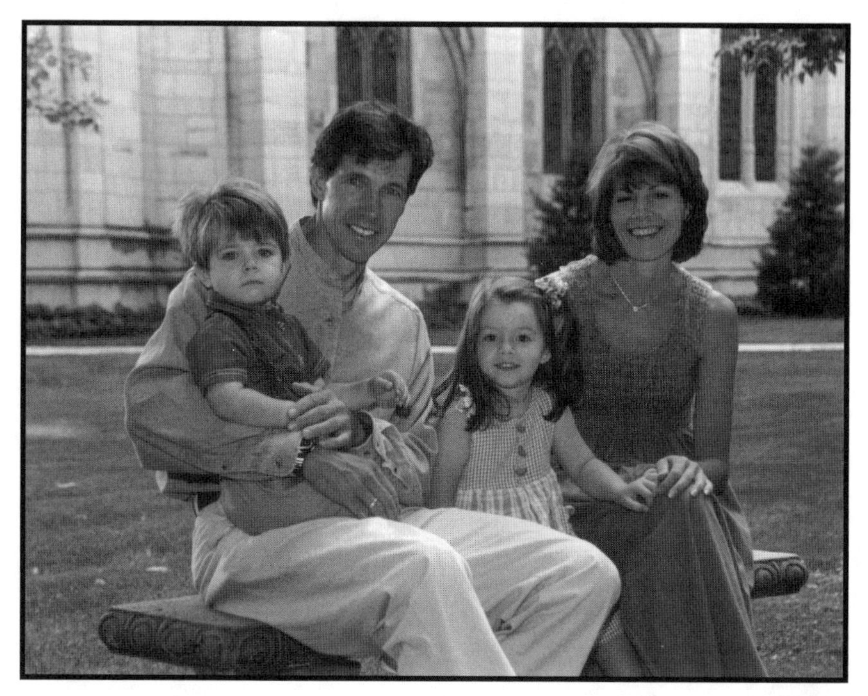

Author Joe Luxbacher and Family

About the Authors

Joe Luxbacher has twenty-five years experience as an athlete, peak performance coach, and physical educator. He holds a PhD in Health, Physical and Recreation Education and is employed in the Department of Athletics at the University of Pittsburgh. Joe has written extensively in the area of sport, fitness, exercise and weight control with 14 books and more than 150 published magazine articles to his credit. Joe is the former fitness editor of *Total Health* Magazine, and presently writes a bi-weekly fitness column for the *Pittsburgh Post-gazette* (400,000 + circulation). Joe lives outside of Pittsburgh, Pennsylvania with his family.

Leslie Bonci is the Director of Sports Medicine Nutrition for the Department of Orthopedic Surgery and the Center for Sports Medicine at the University of Pittsburgh Medical Center. She is a registered dietitian with a Masters' degree is Public Health. Leslie writes regularly for Pennsylvania Health and Fitness magazine, and web sites including Drkoop.com, gymamerica.com, nfl.com and fitnesstimes.com on sports nutrition topics.

Kim King was a pioneer of women's bodybuilding and strength training beginning in 1982, winning numerous national titles after turning professional in 1992. An affiliate of IFBB and NPC, she also judges national and professional fitness and bodybuilding competitions. She has owned and operated fitness center for more than 15 years. She is currently the Head Strength and Conditioning Coach for Olympic Sports at the University of Pittsburgh.